Textbook of Pharmacovigilance

Concept and Practice

Textbook of Pharmacovigilance

Concept and Practice

Guru Prasad Mohanta

M. Pharm., Ph. D.

Prabal Kumar Manna

M . Pharm., Ph. D.

Professors, Department of Pharmacy,
Annamalai University,
Annamalai Nagar – 608 002.

PharmaMed Press

An imprint of Pharma Book Syndicate

A unit of BSP Books Pvt. Ltd.

4-4-309/316, Giriraj Lane,
Sultan Bazar, Hyderabad - 500 095.

Textbook of Pharmacovigilance: ***Concept and Practice by***
Guru Prasad Mohanta and Prabal Kumar Manna

Published by

PharmaMed Press

An imprint of Pharma Book Syndicate

A unit of BSP Books Pvt. Ltd.

4-4-309/316, Giriraj Lane, Sultan Bazar, Hyderabad - 500 095.

Phone: 040-23445605, 23445688; Fax: 91+40-23445611

E-mail: info@pharmamedpress.com

ISBN: 978-93-5230-103-4 (HB)

INDIAN PHARMACOPOEIA COMMISSION
National Coordination Centre, Pharmacovigilance Programme of India
MINISTRY OF HEALTH & FAMILY WELFARE, GOVERNMENT OF INDIA
SECTOR-23, RAJ NAGAR, GHAZIABAD- 201 002.
Tel No: 0120- 6582849, 2783392, 2783400, 2783401; Fax: 2783311
Mail: pvpi@ipcindia.net, Web: www.ipc.gov.in

FOREWORD

Pharmacovigilance has been accepted as an important public health function which aims at reducing the medicine related harms. Intensive efforts are currently ongoing in the country to strengthen the system of Pharmacovigilance Programme of India (PvPI) to ensure the safety of medicines. The PvPI involves a systematic collection of adverse drug reactions (ADRs) data and providing valuable information to drug regulatory authority to take necessary actions in order to promote patients safety.

However, lack of knowledge of where, what and how to report ADRs continue to be the major concern of PvPI. As the entire healthcare professionals are important stakeholders in Pharmacovigilance, it may be more appropriate to educate, train and sensitize them during their course itself on various aspects of Pharmacovigilance.

This book entitled "Textbook of Pharmacovigilance: *Concept and Practice*" provides a unique and valuable resource for learning as well as practicing Pharmacovigilance. I hope the healthcare students and the professionals will find this book of great use to understand the standard definitions, terminologies and other essential elements of Pharmacovigilance. The authors, Dr. Guru Prasad Mohanta and Dr. Prabal Kumar Manna, with their long experience in teaching and reasonable experience in Pharmacovigilance have put their effort in presenting the key principles of Pharmacovigilance in simple language for easy adaptability. Hope the students would find chapters on case studies and global scenario more interesting as they give insight on global activities and scope.

I do hope the book will be used as an important educational intervention tool to promote Pharmacovigilance activities both in health systems and in the industries.

V. Kalaiselvan
Principal Scientific Officer

PREFACE

"There are many who come and go
There are few who leave and mark"

Pharmacovigilance in simplest sense is to "detect the harmful effects of drugs (or medicines) on patients and to reduce the likelihood of their occurrence". This is a new young discipline in Health Sciences but gaining fast acceptance among the health professionals and medicine regulating authorities. India sets to become hub for Pharmacovigilance activities as evident from the large number of IT companies venturing into this area.

Though the subject has lot of relevance in providing quality care to the patients, perhaps there is no regular programme, other than some pharmacy programmes, where the subject is extensively taught. There are few short term courses offered by unorganised sectors. There are very few affordable books too. The authors made a modest attempt to educate and sensitize people who are interested in Pharmacovigilance. While authors are well aware of difficulties writing a textbook on this new emerging science, they are confident in effectively distilling the principles and facts into the present text.

The number, severity and cost of Adverse Drug Reactions (ADRs) have been recognised as a significant public health issue. There has been continuing interest in discovering what causes them and how their occurrences can be predicted or prevented, if feasible. These are the subject matters of the present text. The term drug and medicine have been used interchangeably in the whole text. The authors express their gratitude to the World Health Organization (WHO) for permitting to reproduce some of the materials of WHO in the text. The two chapters, Quality Assurance in Pharmacovigilance and Case Studies on Causality Assessment, are contributed by Mr. Shaikh Ruhu Al Amin and Dr. J. Ponni respectively. These two former students of ours, now successful Pharmacovigilance Professionals, deserve our special appreciation.

We hope the text would help the students and aspiring professionals to acquire the knowledge, necessary skills, and attitudes that would enable them to effectively identify, assess and report ADRs as well as initiate appropriate action besides taking up career in medicine safety programme.

We are grateful to Dr. G. N. Singh, Drugs Controller General of India, for encouragement and gesture of wishing for our effort in developing the text. He is also the Secretary – cum – Scientific Director of Indian Pharmacopoeia Commission and personality responsible for bringing the PV Programme of the Country to such an appreciable level. We are extremely thankful to Dr. V. Kalaiselvan, Principal Scientific Officer at Indian Pharmacopoeia Commission, Government of India, for writing the Foreword for the text. He is the key person coordinating the Pharmacovigilance Programme of India at the National Coordinating Centre (NCC). We appreciate our former student, Dr. Thota Prasad, currently Scientific Assistant at NCC, for extending his expertise throughout the entire period of preparing the text.

We would like to thank the Annamalai University Authorities for permitting us to write the text. We are thankful to our family members for bearing with us during the development of the text. Our PharmD student, Mr. V. Venkatesh, needs a special appreciation for drawing some figures for the book. We express our thanks to Mr. Anil Shah of PharmaMed Press for showing continued interest in publishing the book.

There is nothing more important than hearing the opinion of readers or users of the book. Your opinion matters us and would help us improving the text further to make it more useful.

"Let's act together to make the medicines safer for us and for our next generation as well".

Guru Prasad Mohanta
[gpmohanta@hotmail.com]

Prabal Kumar Manna
[pkmanna@rediffmail.com]

CONTENTS

ABBREVIATIONS

ADR	–	Adverse Drug Reaction
ADRAC	–	Adverse Drug Reaction Advisory Committee
ADROIT	–	ADR Online Information Tracking
AIIMS	–	All India Institute of Medical Sciences
ASU	–	Ayurveda, Siddha and Unani
AYUSH	–	Ayurveda, Yoga and Naturopathy, Unani, Siddha and Homeopathy
BCPNN	–	Bayesian Confidence Propagation Neural Network
BNF	–	British National Formulary
CBER	–	Centre for Biologics Evaluation and Research
CDER	–	Centre for Drug Evaluation and Research
CDSCO	–	Central Drug Standard Control Organization
CEM	–	Cohort Event Monitoring
CIOMS	–	Council for International Organizations of Medical Sciences
COHM/CHM	–	Commission on Human Medicines
CSD	–	Committee on Safety of Drugs
CSM	–	Committee on Safety of Medicines
CT	–	Clinical Trial
DCGI	–	Drugs Controller General of India
DoTS	–	Dose, Time and Susceptibility
EHR	–	Electronic Health Record
EMP	–	Essential Medicines and Health Products
EU	–	European Union
EURD	–	European Union Reference Data
FAERS	–	FDA Adverse Event Reporting System
FDC	–	Food, Drug and Cosmetic
GPvP	–	Good Pharmacovigilance Practice

HIS	–	Health System and Innovation
ICH	–	International Conference on Harmonization
ICMR	–	Indian Council for Medical Research
ICSR	–	Individual Case Safety Report
IPC	–	Indian Pharmacopoeia Commission
ISM	–	Indian System of Medicine
MCC	–	Medicines Control Council
MGPS	–	Multi-item Gamma Poisson Shrinker
MHRA	–	Medicine and Health Products Regulatory Agency
MMR	–	Measles, Mumps and Rubella
MvP	–	Materio Vigilance Programme [Medical Device]
MvPI	–	Materio Vigilance Programme of India
NCC	–	National Coordination Centre
OMSM	–	Office of Medicine Safety Monitoring
PADER	–	Periodic Adverse Drug Experience Report
PAER	–	Periodic Adverse Experience Report
PBRER	–	Periodic Benefit Risk Evaluation Report
PMS	–	Post Marketing Surveillance
PRAC	–	Pharmacovigilance Risk Assessment Committee
PRISM	–	Post-Licensure Rapid Immunization Safety Monitoring Programme
PSUR	–	Periodic Safety Update Report
PV	–	Pharmacovigilance
PvPI	–	Pharmacovigilance Programme of India
QA	–	Quality Assurance
RCT	–	Randomized Control Trial
SDA	–	Signal Detection Algorithm
TGA	–	Therapeutic Good Administration
UMC	–	Uppsala Monitoring Centre
UN	–	United Nations

USA	–	United States of America
USD	–	United States Dollar
USFDA	–	United States Food and Drugs Administration
WHA	–	World Health Assembly
WHO	–	World Health Organization
WHO ART	–	WHO Adverse Reaction Terminology
WHO DD	–	WHO Drug Dictionary
YCS	–	Yellow Card System

Chapter 1

Introduction

"The farther back you look the farther forward you can see"

Winston Churchill

After reading this chapter, you should be able to understand and appreciate:
• The genesis and importance of the term 'Pharmacovigilance'.
• The consequences of Adverse Drug Reactions.
• Historical development of safety monitoring programme.
• The sources of data for Pharmacovigilance.
• Aims of Pharmacovigilance.

Pharmacovigilance is the science of collecting, monitoring, researching, assessing and evaluating information from healthcare providers and patients on the adverse effects of medicines, biological products, herbals and traditional medicines with a view to identify new information about hazards and preventing harm to patients. The word 'Pharmacovigilance' is derived from the Greek word *pharmakon* meaning drug and the Latin word *vigilare* meaning to keep awake or alert, to keep watch. The word was initially used in France in 1960s and later was perceived as the new name for the old terminology post marketing surveillance (PMS). The Pharmacovigilance term is now used internationally. The World Health Organization introduced the term in 2002 and has been adopted by International Conference on Harmonization of Technical Requirements for Registration of Pharmaceuticals for Human Use (ICH). The domain of Pharmacovigilance is not just restricted to PMS but to the entire period of journey of medicines and related products from the pre-approval development to the post approval period.

Safety and efficacy parameters are the prime requirements of evaluation in the process of drug development. While efficacy is important for assessing the usefulness of a testing drug, the safety requirements make it whether to use or not. The possibility that drug use could result in adverse reaction came to the fore rather earlier than did concern about inefficiency. Even, the father of the modern medicine Hippocrates said "Do no harm". There are many quotes which described the importance of safety issues. The two are cited here:

"Cured yesterday of my disease, I died last night of my physician/medicine".

"Go to the Doctor, get your prescription, pay his fees as the doctor has to survive; Go to the Pharmacist, buy your medicine and pay for it, because the pharmacist has to survive; Now go home and throw your medicines because you need to survive".

The quotes are just to emphasize the issues with the use of medicines and they are not to undermine the importance of medicines in everybody's life. The medicines are perhaps the greatest weapon of mankind fighting illnesses, preventing diseases and improving quality of life besides increasing longevity.

The new drugs undergo a significant amount of testing for safety and efficacy in animals and humans through which the effectiveness can be assessed with certainty but the safety issue with less certainty. The clinical trials never tell the whole story of the effects of a drug in all situations. The clinical trials are incomplete studies due to various reasons like limited and selected patients are used; duration of trial is limited; data on special group of patients either not generated or incomplete. The clinical trials can detect only the commonest adverse drug reactions (with more than 1% incidence). The less common adverse drug reactions (with less than 1% incidence) can only be discovered in a long term study in large population. It took decades before the ADRs of Aspirin on gastrointestinal tract became apparent. It also took years to recognise the renal toxicity of phenacetin. This implies the need of continuing drug safety evaluation in post approval period. The safety study in post approval period is also called post marketing surveillance (PMS). The word surveillance is derived from French terms: *sur* (meaning over) and *veiller* (meaning to watch). The terminology post marketing surveillance first appeared in 1960s and is attributed to

Bill Inman, a medically qualified doctor worked in drug safety issues in UK for long time.

Clinical Trials (CT): *They are human experimentations conducted in order to assess the safety and efficacy of prospective drug. CT is broadly divided into: Pre-approval and post approval studies. Pre-approval studies are divided into Phase – I, Phase – II and Phase – III.*

Phase – I: *is conducted in 20-100 healthy volunteers to determine the tolerable concentration, the route of administration and the initial pharmacokinetic information. It also checks the possible side effects.*

Phase – II: *is conducted in 100-500 patients. It provides information on efficacy, short term tolerability and to determine the dose that best balances between efficacy and safety (tolerability).*

Phase – III: *is conducted in 1000-5000 patients to confirm effectiveness and monitor adverse drug reactions from longer use.*

Based on the three phases of studies, the drug is approved for marketing. The post approval studies, also called Phase – IV or Post Marketing Surveillance, are conducted to identify the undiscovered adverse drug reactions.

Consequences of ADRs

Not that all ADRs are very serious but some are definite causes of death, hospitalization, or serious injury. ADRs have two important consequences on the individuals and the health system:

(i) sufferings (including deaths) and prolonged stay at hospital and

(ii) economic impact. ADRs are one of the leading causes of morbidity and mortality.

In USA, 700,000 emergency department visits and 120,000 hospitalizations are due to ADEs annually. USD 3.5 billion is spent on extra medical costs of ADEs annually. At least 40% of costs on ambulatory (non-hospital settings) Adverse Drugs Events management are estimated to be preventable. In UK, some studies showed that the prevalence of hospital admission resulting directly from adverse drug reactions was over 5% and adverse drug reactions accounted for 0.15% of deaths among all admissions. Worldwide on an average 3 to 5% of hospital admissions are attributed to ADRs and 0.32 to 6.7% is the incidence of serious and fatal adverse drug reactions in hospital patients. Due to poor reporting culture much reliable data from India is not available. However, one study from a south Indian hospital [http://www.ncbi.nlm.nih.gov/pubmed/14762985] reported that 3.7% of the hospitalised patients experienced an ADR, 0.7% of the admissions were due to ADRs and 1.8% had a fatal ADR. The average cost of managing an ADR was reported to be Rs. 690/-.

The safety information obtained helps the drug regulating authority to advice on labelling changes to restricting its availability to completely banning the product. Many drugs have been withdrawn from the world market because of actual or perceived safety concern. An estimated one third was withdrawn within two years of launch and a half within five years. Having learnt the importance of safety monitoring of medicines beyond the clinical trials, it may be appropriate to know how the system of safety monitoring has evolved over the years. This is divided into two periods: pre-thalidomide and post thalidomide period.

Pre-Thalidomide Period

The thalidomide disaster changed the world's outlook towards medicines' safety and the world became wiser and started monitoring the medicines in use. This has been a milestone in safety monitoring programme. But there have been records of toxicity caused by the medicines even much before the thalidomide tragedy. Here are few examples of drug safety records that are reported prior to thalidomide: The death of a person during the routine anaesthetic with chloroform in 1848 in north–east England was identified as an episode of ventricular fibrillation. Chloroform was just introduced a year earlier into clinical practice and was known to be better than ether as the former produced less nausea and vomiting. Because of continuing concerns of the public and the profession about the safety of anaesthesia, the Lancet set up a commission which invited doctors in Britain and its colonies to report anaesthesia related deaths. This was viewed as the forerunner of a system of reporting adverse events; the first suspicion that drug might be involved in causing aplastic anaemia was aroused by Labbi and Langlois in 1919 which is around 30 years after the first description of the disease. In 1934, the role of a drug in the aetiology of agranulocytosis was suggested for the first time.

Though the recording or documenting of toxic effects of medicines has a long history, even in USA there was no assurance of safety and effectiveness of medicines till 1930s. The manufacturers were not in obligation to disclose the contents on the label. The legislation of 1906, Pure Food and Drug Act, was meant just to ensure the purity and consistency of food and drugs and also to ensure the clear and accurate identification of active ingredients. The Act was silent on safety and efficacy. Until 1938, the drugs could still be useless and/or dangerous as long as the label listed the ingredients in a correct manner.

Story of Sulfanilamide Elixir: In 1937, a remedy of sore throat called sulfanilamide elixir manufactured by a small factory in Tennessee was found to be the cause of 107 deaths. As the drug was not soluble in water, it was difficult to form a paediatric preparation. The company, ignorant of toxic aspects of the new solvent, dissolved drug in diethelene glycol. The product had not been adequately tested for safety.

USFDA seized the entire stock before causing further deaths. FDA acted not because the drug was not safe. Safety was not an issue as it was not the requirement (1906 regulation). The FDA acted because the preparation had been mislabelled. Technically an elixir had to contain some quantity of ethyl alcohol and it had none. This was in violation of the law.

But the incident made America to make regulation not only to ensure the safety of the drug but of the whole product.

Following the sulfanilamide elixir issue, there was demand for better legislation for ensuring safety or against the unsafe drugs. In December 1937, US Congress passed the legislation that had been stalled for several years. This new legislation called Federal Food, Drug and Cosmetic (FDC) Act had taken effect in 1938. This Act necessitated the requirement of demonstration that new drugs were safe before they could be marketed commercially.

Post-Thalidomide Period

A direct consequence of thalidomide disaster that occurred in several countries outside USA, the US Government had amended the FDC Act, known as Kefeuver–Harris Amendment of 1960. As a result of this amendment, the drug companies were required to prove that new drugs were effective as well as safe. The safety was not a matter of concern till this time. The physicians were instructed through a federal programme called MedWatch to report to the FDA any instance of adverse effect resulting from use of new drug by their patients.

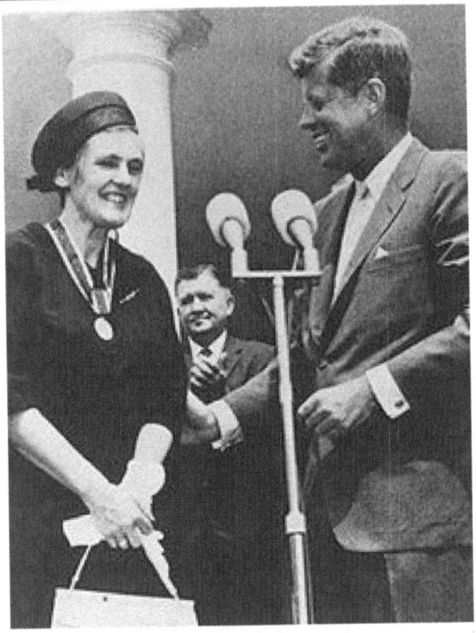

Dr. Frances Kathleen Oldham Kelsey, a pharmacologist in USFDA, prevented the entry of thalidomide into USA market by not approving it. She insisted the need of further studies despite of its approval in UK and other countries. She received commendable appreciation for preventing thalidomide disaster in USA which would have otherwise caused the birth of thousands of armless and legless children. In 1962, she was awarded with President's award for Distinguished Federal Civilian Service from President John F. Kennedy. In 2010 the FDA honoured Kelsey by naming one of their annual awards after her and she was the first recipient.

In UK the Committee on Safety of Drugs (CSD) was formed in 1963. The next year in 1964, it had introduced the Yellow Card system (YCS) with a letter circulated to all doctors urging to report promptly the details of any untoward condition in a patient that might be the result of drug treatment. The YCS is a prepaid system even working today got its name from the colour of the original document used for reporting ADRs. The Medicines and Healthcare Products Regulatory Agency (MHRA) is responsible for ensuring safety and effectiveness of drugs. Committee on Safety of Drugs was replaced by the terminology Committee on Safety of Medicines (CSM) in 1970. Again in 1970, this was replaced by Commission on Human Medicines (CHM).

Again it was felt by World Health Organization (WHO) to have an international system for monitoring adverse reaction to drugs (ADRs) based on the data from national centres. After a pilot study in USA, an international database was established at Geneva, WHO head quarter, in 1971. The base for international monitoring system was moved to Uppsala, Sweden, in 1978. Since then, Uppsala Monitoring Centre (UMC) has been managing the primary aspects of expanding worldwide Pharmacovigilance network of more than 130 countries. UMC is the WHO collaborating Centre for international drug monitoring. India joined the WHO programme in 1998. Currently, India has a very ambitious National Pharmacovigilance Programme with more than 54000 individual case safety reports received by the National coordinating centre located at office of Indian Pharmacopeia Commission [Pharmacovigilance Newsletter, August 2013]. The recent initiative of World Health Organization to make the safety database accessible to all would be helpful promoting safe medications.

Methods in Pharmacovigilance

The Pharmacovigilance data (ADRs reports) comes primarily from spontaneous reporting (also known as volunteering reporting) by the healthcare professionals. This type of reporting is dependent on the initiative and motivation of the potential reporters, the healthcare professionals. These reports are called "individual case safety report (ICSR)". Another issue with the voluntary reporting that doctors may worry that the adverse effects they report may be seen as the result of their bad practice which may not only leave them open to criticism but also to litigation.

In addition to spontaneous reporting of adverse drug reactions, there are systems/methods to have active surveillance. Usually the academic scientists or hospitals or industries contribute significantly by active follow up after treatment. The events may be detected by asking patients directly or screening patients' records. The cohort event monitoring is the most comprehensive method. The active surveillance is also a part of pharmacoepidemiolgy which is defined as the science of investigating the effects of drugs already in the market in large group of population.

Irrespective of the source of data, the reports are analysed for assessing their association with the drug(s) called causality assessment. They are useful in detecting a signal, a notice of an early concern about possible drug safety problem. Detecting signals is one of the primary objectives of Pharmacovigilance. The Pharmacovigilance data provides evidence for making regulatory decisions based on strengthened signals.

Pharmacovigilance Programme aims to:

- Improve patient care through ensuring safety of medicines;
- Improve public health through ensuring safe use of medicines;
- Help in assessment of benefit, harm, effectiveness and risk of medicines;
- Promote understanding, education, and training on Pharmacovigilance to ensure safe use of medicines [Reducing or minimising medicine use related harm].

Conclusion

Pharmacovigilance aims at getting the best outcome from a drug treatment. Though no one wants to harm patients, unfortunately many medicines harm the patients sometimes. Good Pharmacovigilance will identify the risks in the shortest possible time after the medicine is marketed and will help to establish/identify risk factors. The Pharmacovigilance information would allow intelligent and evidence based prescribing with potential for preventing many adverse reactions. This would ultimately ensure optimum therapy at a lowest cost to each patient and the health system.

Dr. Marie Lindquist, Director of Uppsala Monitoring Centre, compares the Pharmacovigilance activities with observational skills of the Sherlock Homes. With his attention to every detail and its meaning and implication help Sherlock to analyze the situation in logical way and solve the mystery. She quotes Sherlock "when you have eliminated the impossible, whatever remains, however improbable, must be the truth".

While the safety of the medicines and the related products are of prime importance to all stake holders: manufacturers, health professionals and the patients, falsely attributing a harmful effect to a medicine, or a treatment, causes a lot of damage which can be difficult to reverse. The reported causal relationship between the MMR (Measles, Mumps and Rubella) vaccination and autism influenced the patients rejecting the vaccine. MMR vaccine was introduced in UK in 1988 as a replacement of individual vaccines. Following the study reported in the Lancet in 1998 on the possible link between the autism and MMR vaccine raised an alarm among the parents. This impacted the higher prevalence of measles in the UK. There were 2,016 confirmed cases of measles in England and Wales in 2012, the highest total for 18 years. However, One of the biggest studies of all - a 2002 paper examining the records of 537,303 children born in Denmark - also showed no link between MMR and autism [http://www.bbc.co.uk/news/health-22173393 accessed on 19 October 2013].

Key Messages

- The word 'pharmacovigilance' is originated in France in 1960 from Greek word 'pharmakon' [meaning drug] and Latin word 'vigilare' [meaning to keep watch].
- Though pharmacovigilance originally intended for safety monitoring of approved medicines (post-marketing surveillance), now it includes the safety monitoring for the entire period of life cycle inclusive of pre- approval and post- approval period.
- Pre-approval clinical trials cannot detect all adverse drug reactions but only the common ones with more than 1% incidence. Hence, there is a need of post-marketing surveillance when medicines are used by large section of the population.
- Though all adverse drug reactions are equally harmful affecting human health, they are one of the leading causes of morbidity and mortality worldwide.
- Safety information (Adverse drug reaction reports) collected in pharmacovigilance programme helps the regulatory authority (Government) to take appropriate action ranging from advices on labelling change to restricting availability to completely banning a product.
- Following Thalidomide disaster of 1960s the countries had initiated programme on safety monitoring including the International drug monitoring by WHO. At present 130 countries are participating in WHO's programme.
- India's National Pharmacovigilance Programme is coordinated by Indian Pharmacopoeia Commission.
- Pharmacovigilance aims to ensure safe and optimum therapy.

Bibliography

1. View Point – Part 1, the Uppsala Monitoring Centre, 2002.
2. View Point – Part 2, the Uppsala Monitoring Centre, 2005.
3. Safety of Medicines, World Health Organization, Geneva, 2002.
4. The Importance of Pharmacovigilance, World Health Organization, 2002.
5. Guru Prasad Mohanta, Textbook on Clinical Research: A Guide for Aspiring Professionals and Professionals, PharmaMed Press, 2001.
6. Management of Safety Information from Clinical Trials, Report of CIOMS Working Group VI, CIOMS, Geneva, 2005.
7. MNG Dukes, Drug Utilization Studies, WHO Regional Publications, 1993.

Chapter 2

Pharmacovigilance in India

"The worst thing about medicine is that one kind makes another necessary".

Elbert Hubbard

After reading this chapter, you should be able to understand and appreciate:
• The need and genesis of pharmacovigilance programme in India. • The salient features of National Pharmacovigilance Programme [World Bank Project]. • The salient features of Pharmacovigilance Programme of India [Currently in Operation]. • The functioning of Pharmacovigilance Programme of India. • The basics of related programmes: Materiovigilance, Haemovigilance and Vaccine Pharmacovigilance.

The Indian Pharmaceutical Industries have made tremendous progress in terms of infrastructure development, technology base and wide range of products in last few decades. The strength of Indian pharmaceutical industries is in developing cost effective technologies in shortest possible time without compromising qualities. Many of the Indian companies have international regulatory approvals for their plants from agencies like USFDA, MHRA-UK, TGA-Australia, MCC – South Africa etc. The country exports medicines to more than 200 countries including USA, Canada, UK, etc. In fact, the whole world looks for India for cost-effective generic medicines. India is known as Pharmacy of Third World. It is the third largest in the world in terms of volume and 14th in terms of value accounting for around 10% of world's production by volume and 1.5% by value.

India becomes a favourite clinical research destination as there has been increasing focus on cost cutting in drug development process. Clinical trials seem to be 10-50% cheaper in India compared to the cost involved in developed countries. The booming clinical research in India is evident from India's apex drug regulatory authority's (Central Drug Standard Control Organization) statistics. The number of new Drug Application has increased to 1753 in 2009 from 1200 in 2005. The global clinical trials' number is increased from 100 in 2005 to 262 in 2009 with a peak of 350 in 2008. Safety monitoring of test products during the clinical trials or clinical research is an important requirement. Besides, many new products too are approved for use in India. The safety monitoring of introduced new drugs is mandatory as post marketing surveillance.

The growth of Indian pharmaceutical industries together with rapid growth of clinical research scenario emphasizes the need of a robust safety monitoring programme, Pharmacovigilance Programme. Realising the need of such programme, the Government of India re-launched the massive and ambitious National Pharmacovigilance Programme in 2010 with its own expense. The earlier National Programme was initiated in 2004 with World Bank assistance that stopped functioning in 2008 as the project ended.

Every country needs to have its own Pharmacovigilance programme not just relies on the International Programme as there are Geographical differences in disease prevalence, Genetic Polymorphism, Healthcare system, Healthcare practices, Indications for use of medicines, Formulation practices and Drug use monitoring practices.

The ADR monitoring programme is not new to India though not much progress has been made. In 1982, five centres were established by the Drugs Controller of India. Indian Council for Medical Research (ICMR) had collected about 58,000 reports through its multi-institutional study but they all stopped functioning after few years. In 1989, six regional centres were set up in Bombay, New Delhi, Calcutta, Lucknow, Pondicherry and Chandigarh under the aegis of Drugs Controller of India. In 1987, the India finally joined the WHO ADR monitoring programme with Department of Pharmacology, All India Institute of Medical Sciences (AIIMS) as National Centre and KEM hospital (Bombay) and

JLN Hospital, Aligarh Muslim University, Aligarh, as the WHO special centres. These centres and the programme could not be sustained due to lack of adequate funding and other factors.

World bank funded national pharmacovigilance programme: Realizing the need of vibrant Pharmacovigilance programme in the country to protect the population from the potential harm that may be caused by use of new drugs (in the backdrop of new product patent regime from 2005, it was expected of large scale clinical trials in India), the central drugs control authority proposed the setting up of Pharmacovigilance programme in 2004. With commitment of USD 1,00,000 from World Bank assisted capacity building project, the Central Drugs Standard Control Organization (CDSCO) launched the National Pharmacovigilance Programme in November 2004. Mr. Brigesh Regal, the then WHO Consultant to DCGI, was instrumental in drafting the whole programme and the then Health Minister, Dr. Anbumani Ramadoss, launched the programme in New Delhi on 23 November 2004.

The programme was based on the recommendations made in WHO publication entitled "Safety Monitoring of Medicinal Products – Guidelines for Setting Up and Running a Pharmacovigilance Centre". The National Pharmacovigilance Advisory Committee (NPAC) was constituted under the chairmanship of Director General of Health Services to oversee the performance of various centres and recommend possible regulatory measures based on data received from various centres. The NPAC consisted of:

1. Chairman, Director General of Health Services.
2. Member Secretary, DCG(I).
3. ICMR D. G., ICMR, New Delhi.
4. Ministry of Health and Family Welfare, Director I/c of Drugs Division.
5. AIIMS, New Delhi, Zonal Centre Coordinator, Dr. S.K. Gupta, Head of the Department, Pharmacology, AIIMS, New Delhi
6. SGC Medical College, Mumbai, Zonal Centre Coordinator, Dr. Nilima Kshirsagar, SGS, Medical College, (Mumbai)
7. Member, Pharmacology: Dr. Ranjit Roy Chaudhary, NII, New Delhi and Dr. C. Adithan, Prof. Pharmacology, JIPMER, Pondicherry.

8. Member, Forensic Medicine: Dr. T.D. Dogra, AIIMS, New Delhi.
9. Member, General Medicine: Dr. Anoop Mishra (AIIMS, New Delhi) and Dr. A.K. Agarwal (RML, New Delhi).
10. Member, Clinical Pharmacology: Dr. S.D. Seth, Chair-in Clinical Pharmacology (ICMR, New Delhi).
11. Member, Pharmacy: Mr. Brijesh Regal, Former WHO Consultant (New Delhi).
12. Member, Toxicology: Dr. Y.K. Gupta, Director, (ITRC, Lucknow).
13. Member, Epidemiology: Dr. M.D. Gupte (ICMR Institute of Epidemiology, Chennai).
14. Member, Pathology: Dr. Kusum Verma, Member Secretary, (AIIMS Ethics Committee, New Delhi).
15. Member, Drug Information: Dr. Pramil Tiwari (NIPER, Mohali).
16. Member, Phytotherapy: Dr. Urmila Thatte, Head of the Department, Pharmacology, B. L. Nair, Medical College Hospital, Mumbai.

The National Programme was launched with the aims to:

I. Contribute to the regulatory assessment of benefit, harm, effectiveness and risk of medicines, encouraging their safe, rational and more effective (including cost effective) use.
II. Improve patient care and safety in relation to use of medicines and all medicinal and paramedical interventions.
III. Improve public health and safety in relation to use of medicines.
IV. Promote understanding, education and clinical training in Pharmacovigilance and its effective communications to the public.

For the purpose of the programme, the whole country was divided into zones and regions for operational efficiency. CDSCO was the main coordinating centre (latter shifted to Department of Pharmacology, AIIMS, New Delhi). It had two zonal centres, five regional centres and twenty eight peripheral centres.

The programme was intended to achieve three broad objectives: short term objective was to foster a reporting culture; the intermediate objective was to involve large number of healthcare professionals in the system in information dissemination; and the long term objective was for the programme to be a benchmark for global drug monitoring.

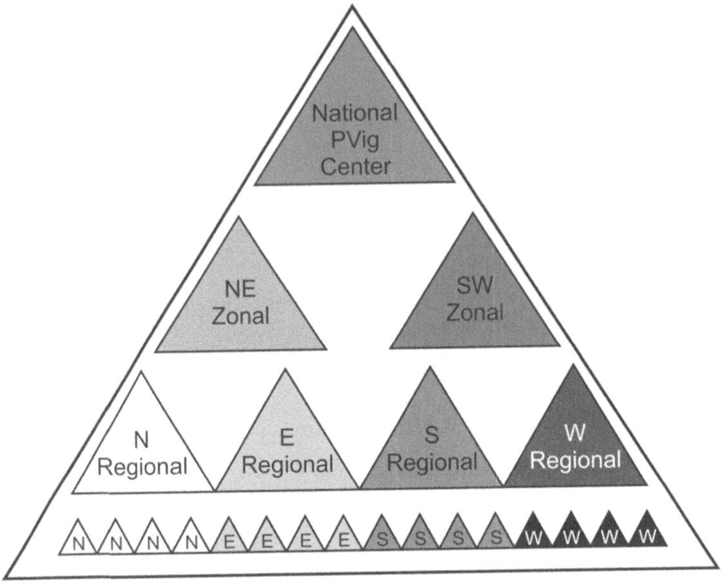

Structure of National Pharmacovigilance Programme

The important terms and responsibilities of various types of centres were:

Parameters	Peripheral Centre	Regional Centre	Zonal Centre
Status	Primary PV Centre	Secondary PV Centre	Tertiary PV Centre
Duration	04 years with a review at the end of every year	04 years with a review at the end of every year	04 years with a review at the end of every year
Primary Task	1. Collect and collate minimum 30 Adverse Drug Event notifications per month and forward all duly filled forms to the assigned regional centre. 2. Carry out special project on drug safety at the request of CDSCO.	1. Correspond with peripheral centres, provide them technical support, coordinate and monitor their functioning. 2. Collect and collate Adverse Events notifications from peri-pheral as well as own centre and forward all duly filled forms to the respective zonal centre.	1. Interact with regional centres and provide them technical support, coordinate and monitor their functions. 2. Collect, collate and computerize the data reported by the regional centres and by its own centre.

Contd...

Parameters	Peripheral Centre	Regional Centre	Zonal Centre
	3. Carry out (and/or review) data causality analysis of all Adverse Drug Events.	3. Ensure quality of data reported by peripheral centres by carrying out technical audits to ensure compliance, take corrective measures and monitor the implementation of corrective measures. 4. Carry out special projects on drug safety at the request for CDSCO. 5. Carry out (and/or review) data causality analysis of all Adverse Drug Events. **6.** 50 Adverse Drug Event notification forms to be collected per month.	3. Monitor quality of data reported by regional and peripheral centres by carrying out technical audits to ensure compliance, take corrective measures and ensure implementation of corrective measures. 4. Carry out special project on drug safety at the request of CDSCO. 5. Carry out (and/or review) data causality analysis of all Adverse Drug Events. 6. Review the account statement received from regional centres and submit audited statement of expenditure within three months completion of financial year. **7.** 100 Adverse Drug Event notification forms to be collected per month.
Support from the Project	No manpower support. Office operation of Rs. 15,000 per annum was provided.	One Technical staff was provided: Pharmacologist [M. Pharm. with pharmacology or Clinical Pharmacy] with remuneration of Rs. 15,000/- per month. Office operation of Rs. 25,000 per annum was provided.	One Technical staff and one Computer Data Operator were provided: Technical Staff Pharmacologist [M. Pharm. with pharmacology or Clinical Pharmacy] with remuneration of Rs. 15,000/- per month. Computer Operator or

Contd...

Parameters	Peripheral Centre	Regional Centre	Zonal Centre
			Data Manager: Graduate with at least one year computer diploma and experience in data handling and up-dation. Office operation of Rs. 25,000 per annum was provided.

Though there were lot of enthusiasm in the beginning, this could not be sustained. There was no full time staff at CDSCO to look after the programme. Even WHO Country Office wanted to support a full time expert to CDSCO, but could not materialize. The outcome or output of the programme was not encouraging. There was lack of communication from top to the bottom in the structure, flow of fund often was the issue and there were other reasons too. This was the first structured programme with prescribed tasks for each centre with monitoring provisions. However, the merit of the programme was that it had centres from private community pharmacy to pharmacy colleges (with pharmacy practice programme) and medical colleges. The new programme launched later in 2010, at least beginning phase, concentrated only on medical colleges as centres.

Pharmacovigilance Programme of India (PvPI)

Post 2005 there has been tremendous increase in number of applications relating to new chemical entity and their approval by drugs regulatory authority. This is reflected from the CDSCO data: 10,000 applications in 2005 to 22,806 in 2009. The rapid induction of new drugs and high tech pharmaceutical products to the health care market threw new challenges and this necessitates the need of a nationwide programme to monitor adverse drug reactions. As the World Bank Project ended, the government of India planned to restart the National Pharmacovigilance Programme. With this in mind, a brain storming workshop was organized in the Department of Pharmacology, All India Institute of Medical Sciences (AIIMS) in 2009 in association with CDSCO and WHO Country office for India. This meeting formulated the frame work of the new programme and was operational from mid July 2010. The CDSCO initiated this new PvPI 14 July 2010 with Department of Pharmacology, AIIMS, New Delhi, as the National Co-Ordination Centre. The National Co-Ordination Centre (NCC) has been shifted to Indian Pharmacopoeia

Commission, Ghaziabad with effect from 15 April 2011. The NCC operates under the supervision of Steering Committee to recommend procedures and guidelines for regulatory interventions.

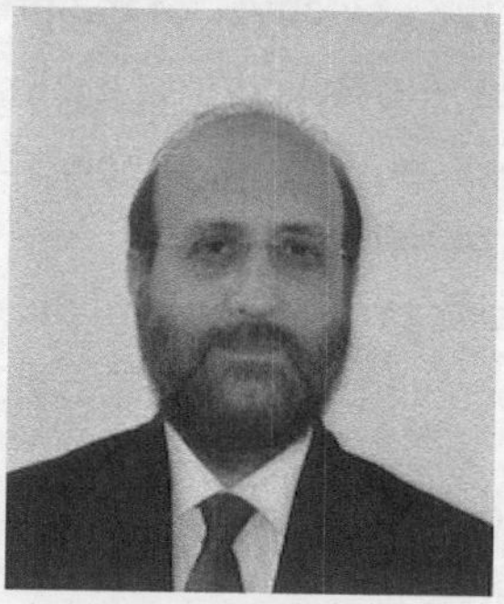

Dr Surinder Singh, Former Drugs Controller General (India), was responsible for re-launching the National Pharmacovigilance Programme in India in 2010 with its own budgetary support. He is also responsible for initiating National Haemovigilance Programme in 2012. Currently Dr. Singh is the Director of National Institute of Biologicals, Government of India.

Supervision

The Steering Committee is consisting of DCGI as *ex-officio* Chairman and Officer in Charge (New Drugs), CDSCO, as *ex-officio* Secretary. In addition it has another 8 members:

1. Scientific Director, Indian Pharmacopoeia Commission, Ghaziabad, *Ex- Officio*,
2. Head, Department of Pharmacology, AIIMS, *Ex- Officio*,
3. Nominee of Director General, Indian Council for Medical Research, *Ex- Officio*,
4. Assistant Director General, Extended Programme of Immunization, as representative of Directorate General of Health Services,
5. Under Secretary (Drugs Control) as representative of the Ministry of Health and Family Welfare,
6. Nominee of Vice Chancellor of Medical / Pharmacy University, *Ex- Officio*,
7. Nominee of Medical Council of India, *Ex- Officio*,
8. Nominee of Pharmacy Council of India, *Ex- Officio*.

Goal and Objectives

The goal of the new programme is to safeguard the health of Indian population through ensuring benefits of medicine use outweighing the risks. The followings are the objectives of the programme:

- To monitor Adverse Drug Reactions (ADRs) in Indian Population.
- To create awareness among healthcare professionals about the importance of ADR reporting in India.
- To monitor benefit-risk profile of medicines.
- To generate independent, evidence based recommendations on safety of medicines.
- To support the CDSCO for formulating safety related regulatory decisions for medicines.
- To communicate finding to all key stakeholders.
- To create a National Centre of Excellence on par with global drug safety monitoring standards.

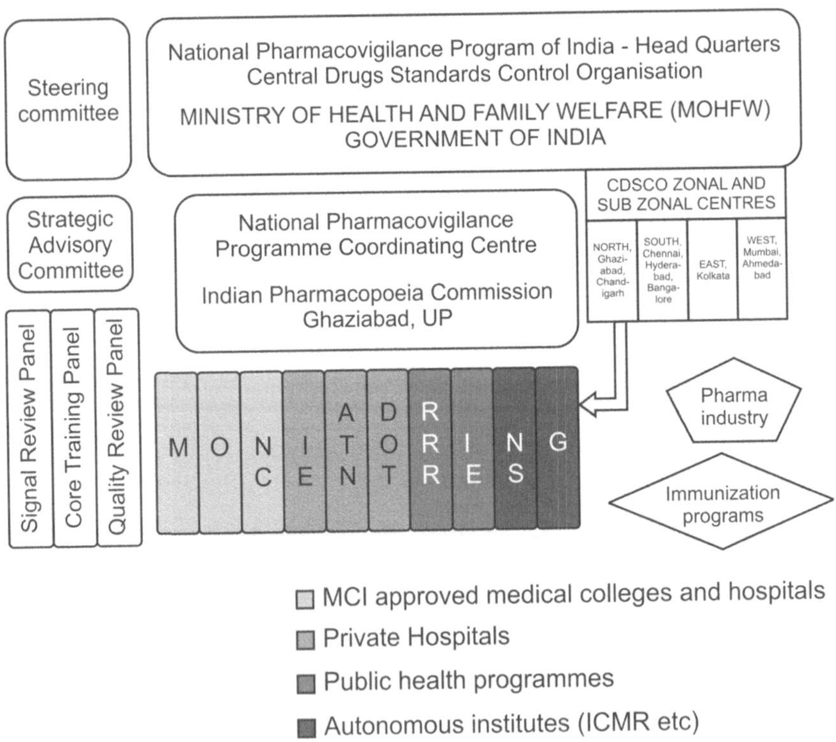

Road Map and Target

The five year road map of the programme (2010 to 2015) has fixed the following targets to achieve:

Period (Phase)	Targets
2010-2011 (Initiation Phase)	Developing systems and procedures. Enrol 40 medical colleges. Start data collection from Adverse Events Following Immunization (AEFI). Development and establishment of training centres. Training of Pharmacovigilance human resource. Linkage with Uppsala Monitoring Centre, Sweden (WHO Collaborating Centre). Initiate software development for National Drug Safety Data Base. Zonal workshops for public awareness of drug safety. Publication of Drug Safety Newsletter.
2011-2012 (Expansion and Consolidation Phase)	Enrol 60 additional medical colleges. Training of Pharmacovigilance human resource. Identify gaps and address through appropriate training. Training on Pharmacovigilance software provided by Uppsala Monitoring Centre (Vigiflow). Software development and validation. Zonal workshops for public awareness of drug safety. Publication of Drug Safety Newsletter.
2012-2013 (Expansion and Maintenance Phase)	Enrol additional 100 medical colleges. Training of Pharmacovigilance human resource. Zonal workshops for public awareness of drug safety. Publication of Drug Safety Newsletter.
2013-2014 (Expansion and Optimization Phase)	Enrol additional 100 medical colleges. Interaction with International Pharmacovigilance Bodies. Training of Pharmacovigilance human resource. Publication of Drug Safety Newsletter.
Excellence Phase (2014-2015)	Create Centre of Excellence for Pharmacovigilance in Asia Pacific.

Operational Principles and Responsibilities of Centres

I. ***Centres:*** Medical Council of India approved Medical College Hospitals, Private Hospitals, Public Health Programmes and Autonomous Institutes like ICMR are planned to be enrolled as ADR monitoring centres. It is proposed to enrol 300 centres by the end of the five year period.

The medical college centres enrolled under the programme are provided technical, administrative, and financial support by the respective zonal / sub-zonal CDSCO office.

The autonomous institutes/other medical institutes/central institutes are planned to be enrolled on voluntary basis but are not provided any support from CDSCO. Similarly public as well as corporate hospitals are also planned for enrolment on voluntary basis but without any support from CDSCO.

II. *Responsibilities:*

Centre	Functions
Medical College ADR Monitoring Centre	• Collection of ADR reports. • Perform follow up with the complainant to check completeness and as per SOP. • Data entry into Vigiflow. • Reporting to National Coordinating Centre through Vigiflow with the source data (original) attached with each ADR case. • Training / Sensitization / Feedback to physicians through Newsletter circulated by the NCC.
Other Centres (Corporate Hospitals, Autonomous Institutes, Pharmaceutical Industry, Public Health Programmes)	• Collection of ADR reports. • Perform follow up with the complainant to check completeness as per SOP. • Report the data to CDSCO Head Quarter.
National Coordinating Centre, IPC, Ghaziabad	• Preparation of SOPs, guidance documents and training manuals. • Data collation, Cross check completeness, Causality Assessment etc. as per SOPs. • Conduct training workshops for all enrolled centres. • Publication medicines safety Newsletter. • Reporting to CDSCO HQ. • Analysis of PMS, PSUR, AEFI data received from CDSCO HQ.
Zonal / Sub-Zonal CDSCO Offices	• Provide procurement, financial and administrative support to ADR monitoring centres. • Report to CDSCO HQ.
CDSCO HQ, New Delhi	• Take appropriate regulatory decision and action on the basis of recommendation of NCC (IPC, Ghaziabad).

Contd...

Centre	Functions
	• Propagation of medicine safety related decisions to stakeholders. • Collaboration with WHO Centre at Uppsala. • Provide for budgetary provisions and administrative support to run Pharmacovigilance Programme.

III. *Monitoring and Evaluation*:

The programme has identified the various indicators to measure the efficiency of process, outcomes and impact of the programme:

Process indicators

- Number of ADR monitoring centres participating in the programme.
- Number of ADR Monitoring Centre trained in a year.
- Funds budgeted and spent.
- Number of ADR Monitoring Centre Personnel working full time for the programme.

Outcome indicators

- Software platform established.
- Number of ADR reports received in a year.
- Number of ADR reports processed in a year.
- Number of ADR reports submitted to Vigiflow.

Impact indicators

- Number of signals generated and confirmed.
- Number of safety related alerts issued by CDSCO.

The PvPI supports professional staff, designated Technical Associate, to each of the medical college centres with consolidated salary of Rs. 20,000/- per month. The qualification prescribed for Technical Associate are: MBBS / MD in Microbiology / Biochemistry / Pharmacology; or Post Graduate in Biochemistry / Microbiology / Biotechnology / Pharmacy.

At present (early 2015), the programme has 150 adverse drug monitoring centres. India has the distinction of reporting over one lakh individual case safety reports (ICSRs) to international database and India is currently the 7th largest contributor to the UMC's international drug safety database (Vigibase) with completeness score of 0.94 out of 1 assessed for Indian ICSRs. A copy of the Adverse Drug Reaction Reporting Form is available in Appendix. In order to encourage the reporter, the Indian Pharmacopoeia Commission, the NCC, has introduced the SMS acknowledgement service through a toll free helpline number: 1800 180 3024. The helpline number is available between 9.00 AM to 5.30 PM on Weekdays.

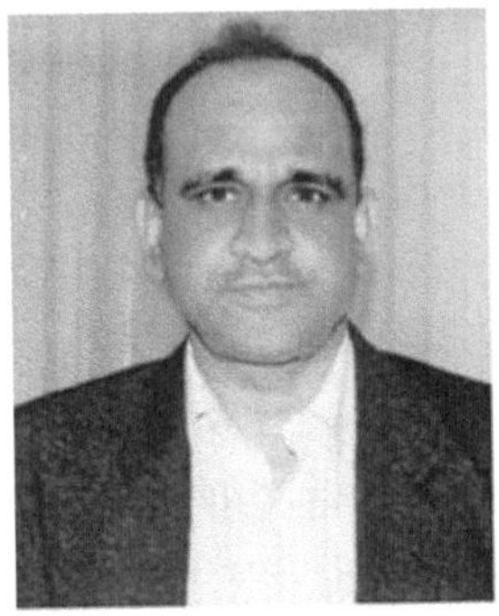

As a Secretary cum Scientific Director, Indian Pharmacopoeia Commission, Government of India, Dr. G. N. Singh was instrumental in strengthening the re-launched National Pharmacovigilance Programme. With his initiative National Coordinating Centre is shifted to the office of Indian Pharmacopoeia Commission, Ghaziabad. He is also the Drugs Controller General (India).

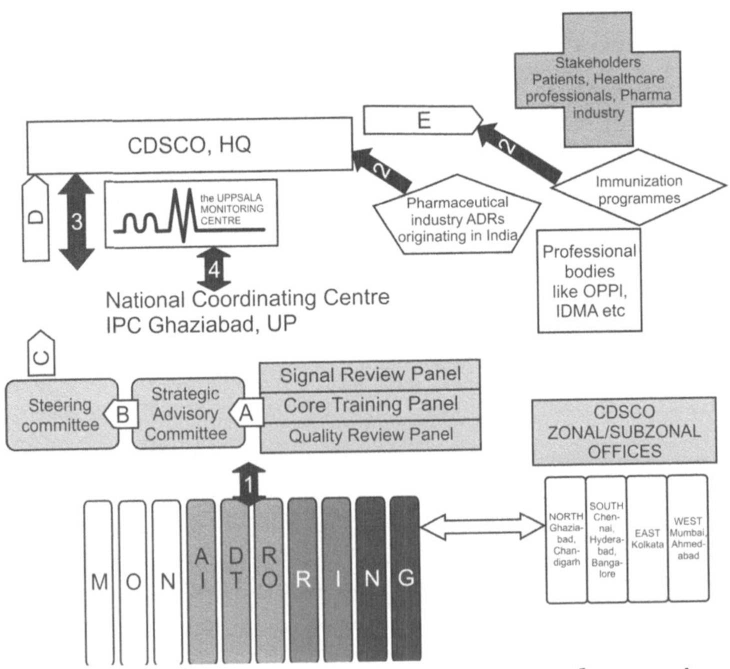

[Source: cdsco.nic.in]

List of Drugs Banned from 2004 onwards	Warning or Other Regulatory Measures taken 2004 onwards

1. Rofecoxib and its formulations (2004)
2. Valdecoxib and its formulations (2005).
3. Diclofenac and its formulations (for Animal Use) (2008).
4. Rimonabant (2009).
5. Rosiglitazone (2010).
6. Nimesulide formulations for chidren below 12 years (2011).
7. Cisapride and its formulations (2011).
8. Phenypropanolamine and its formulations for human use (2011) (Matter in Court).
9. Human Placental Extract and its formulations for human use except its
  1. Topical application for wound healing, and
  2. Injection for pelvic inflame-matory disease. (2011).
10. Sibutramine and its formulations (2011).
11. R-Sibutramine and its formulations (2011).
12. Gatifloxacin formulation for systemic use including oral and injectables but excluding ophthalmic products (2011).
13. Tegaserod and its formulations (2011).
14. Letrozole for induction of ovulation in anovulatory infertility (2011)
15. Analgin (2013) [it is reintroduced with labelling change].
16. Dextyropropoxyphene (2013)
	1. Acetaminophen (Paracetamol) Combination Products:
	• Limiting the prescription combination products: limiting 325 mg.
	• Box Warning: Taking more than daily dose may cause serious liver damage or allergic reactions (e.g. swelling of the face, mouth and throat, difficulty in breathing, itching or rash) (2011).
	2. Artemisinin single therapy manufacturing cancelled (2011).
	3. Box Warning: Use of Nimesulide should ordinarily be restricted to 10 days. If longer clinical use is warranted, liver function tests should be assessed periodically (2012).
	4. Statins Labelling Changes – removing the routine liver function monitoring, inclusion of side effects like memory loss, confusion, hyperglycemia, etc.
	5. Serodiagnostic test kits for diagnosis of Tuberculosis manufacturing License cancelled and the products recalled (2012).
	6. Directing the importer or manufacturers to submit or update the PSUR of new drugs on prescribed format (2012).

The Parliamentary Standing Committee felt that the conventional system of identifying side effects through spontaneous reporting by doctors to either drug companies or drug regulators has been found to be unsatisfactory. It said in the report and recommendation to the Ministry of Health and Family Welfare "The most effective system is by controlled post – marketing (Phase IV) studies on a very large number of patients. In the past decade, all the major adverse effects that led to banning of drugs were identified in large scale Phase – IV trials. The Ministry may wish to consider the possibility of using this format in the country". This observation has made to change the functioning of CDSCO and keeps one of the goals is to protect the public health. The current regulation requires mandatory submission of periodic safety update reports (PSUR) for all new drugs to CDSCO every six months for the first two years of launching the product and annually for the next two years. The very few companies comply with this mandatory requirement and same was reflected in Parliamentary Committee report. Now the Government initiates a process of integrating PSUR submitted by the companies with PvPI. This would further strengthen the safety monitoring programme as PvPI would be able to analyse the PSURs.

In another new initiative, the National Coordinating Centre, IPC, launched the Android Mobile Application in association with NSCB Medical College, Jabalpur, to further strengthening the National Programme. The application has very interesting in built features which would help the private healthcare professionals to report the adverse events in a simple way.

Several software companies too have ventured into pharmacovigilance and this has increased the skilled manpower requirement for carrying out pharmacovigilance activities ranging from basic case processing to complex functions such as signal detection and analysis. Perhaps India would be favourable destination for global pharmacovigilance activities.

Other Programmes

Adverse events monitoring for medical devices: Realizing the need of adverse events monitoring the Government of India now approved a programme called Materio Vigilance Programme [MvP] in an effort to ensure safety of medical devices. Like Pharmacovigilance Programme of India, this nationwide programme called, Materio Vigilance Programme of India (MvPI) is proposed to be coordinated by the Indian Pharmacopeia Commission. The programme intends to monitor medical device associated adverse events (MDAE), create awareness among health professionals about the importance of MDAE reporting and to monitor the benefit –risk profile of medical devices. It is also meant to generate independent evidence based recommendations on the safety of medical devices and to communicate the findings to all stakeholders.

The biotechnology wing of the Sree Chitra Thirunal Institute of Medical Sciences and Technology in Thiruvananthapuram is to be designated as the national collaborating centre for the programme. With Government funding, to begin with it is proposed to establish MvPI cells in 10 Medical colleges.

Haemovigilance programme of india (HvPI): Haemovigilance is a continuous process of data collection and analysis of transfusion related adverse reactions in order to investigate their causes and outcomes and prevent their occurrence or reoccurrences. This nationwide HvPI is launched by Indian Pharmacopoeia Commission in association with National Institute of Biologicals. The programme was launched on 10th December 2012 in already enrolled medical colleges under pharmacovigilance programme of India. National Institute of Biologicals (NIB) is designated as coordinating centre to collate and analyse data with respect to adverse reactions/ events associated with blood transfusion and blood products administration.

Through the use of Haemovigilance Transfusion Reaction Reporting Form (TRRF) and Haemovigil Software, the progrmame is managed. The website for the programme: http://www.nib.gov.in/haemovigilance.html

Vaccine pharmacovigilance: Vaccines and vaccinations are one of the best medical interventions in medical sciences for promoting public health. Ever since the success of small pox vaccine eradicating the dreaded smallpox from the world, the immunization programmes strengthened worldwide including India to prevent preventable diseases. The Government of India in December 2014 launched 'Mission Indradhanush' to achieve complete immunization for all children by 2020 against seven diseases: diphtheria, whooping cough, tetanus, polio, TB, measles and hepatitis B.

The vaccines are different from other medicinal products. The other medicinal products are meant for patients while the vaccines are basically meant for healthy persons mostly children. Realizing the safety concern of vaccines, the Indian regulation keeps the vaccines as new drugs while all other medicinal products (drugs) are treated as new drugs only for four years of their introduction to market or entry into pharmacopoeia whichever is earlier. The death of even one child during immunization practice not only causes grave psychological issues in the mind of vaccinator, it also threatens the very foundation of basis of immunization. The community looses trust.

The safety monitoring of vaccines is essential like that of other medicinal products. The vaccine pharmacovigilance is defined as the science and activities relating to detection, assessment, understanding, prevention and communication of adverse events following immunization or any other vaccine or immunization related issues. The India's programme is known as 'Adverse Event Following Immunization (AEFI)' Surveillance and Response. The safety of vaccines or AEFI Surveillance system was initiated in 1986 and is monitored by the Division of Adverse Events Following Immunization (AEFI), Ministry of Health and Family Welfare. The goals of AEFI Surveillance are to: minimize the negative impact of AEFI on public health, monitor the quality of vaccine used for immunization, ensure and monitor the quality of immunization services, and reduce morbidity and mortality due to AEFIs.

AEFI is a medical incident that takes place after an immunization causes concern and is believed to have caused by immunization. The details of AEFI are available in Government of India's AEFI Surveillance and Response-Operational Guidelines. The responsibility of reporting depends on the site of vaccination: It is Auxiliary Nurse Midwife (ANM) and medical officers in rural areas; and health workers and medical officers in urban areas. The private practitioners both in rural and urban areas who administer vaccines need to report to the District Health Authority. There are two channels of reporting: Monthly Routine Reporting and immediate serious AEFI reporting. All serious AEFI are to be immediately notified by the first person who identifies the event. The first person should notify the case to the nearest Government Primary Health Centre, Community Health Centre, and /or District Immunization Officer by quickest means of communication.

With collaboration of AEFI Surveillance and Pharmacovigilance Programme of India (PvPI), a reporter can report AEFI cases either to Adverse Drug Reaction Monitoring Centre (AMC) or National Coordinating Centre (NCC). This is an additional method of reporting. The AEFI cases reported to PvPI are further coordinated with National level AEFI Committee and State Expanded Programme Immunization Officers for reporting and investigation.

Key Messages

- India is a favourite destination for conducting clinical trials and source of cost effective medicines. It exports medicines to more than 200 countries. With increasing regulatory requirements globally India has the obligation to have its own medicine safety monitoring programme and not just dependent of international programmes. There are geographical differences in Disease prevalence, Genetic polymorphism, Healthcare system, Healthcare practices, Indications for use of medicines, Formulation practices and Drug use monitoring practices. This necessitated the need of National Programme on Pharmacovigilance.
- Central Drug Standard Control Organisation (CDSCO) is the apex body responsible for safety monitoring programme of medicines.
- Though first initiative of ADR monitoring was made in 1982, the first Nationwide Pharmacovigilance Programme was launched during November 2004 under a capacity building project funded by World Bank. The programme ended in 2008 as the funding stopped. There were lot of concerns too on the outcome of the programme. The programme was structured but failed to make an impact mostly due to poor coordination.
- The National Programme is re-launched as 'Pharmacovigilance Programme of India' in July 2010. Now the programme has budgetary support for sustainability and about 150 ADR Monitoring Centres. During the short period, it achieved the distinction of reporting of more than one lakh individual case safety reports to Uppsala's International Drug Monitoring Database besides good quality of report. Indian Pharmacopoeia Commission is the National Coordination Centre.
- The country has similar programmes for medical devices (materio vigilance), blood and blood products (haemovigilance) and vaccines (AEFI Surveillance).

Bibliography

1. J. Vijay Venkataraman, Current Status of Pharmacovigilance in India, Pharmabiz, 1st April 2015.
2. C. Adithan, National Pharmacovigilance Programme, Indian Journal of Pharmacology (editorial), December 2005.
3. Y. K. Gupta, Ensuring Patient Safety – Launching the New Pharmacovigilance Programme of India, Pharma Times, August 2010.
4. http://cdsco.nic.in/html/pharmaco.html accessed on 02 September 2012.
5. www.cdsco.nic.in accessed on 02 September 2012.
6. http://ipc.nic.in/index1.asp?linkid=222 accessed on 02 September 2012.

7. Pipasha Biswas and Arun K Biswas, Setting standards for proactive Pharmacovigilance in India: The way forward, Indian Journal of Pharmacology, June 2007.
8. Department Related Parliamentary Standing Committee on Health and Family Welfare, 59th Report on the Functioning of the CDSCO, May 2012.
9. AEFI Surveillance and Response, Operational Guidelines, Government of India, 2010.

Chapter 3

Methods in Pharmacovigilance

"Whatever you do will be insignificant, but it is very important that you do it".

Mahatma Gandhi

After reading this chapter, you should be able to understand and appreciate:
• Concept of active Pharmacovigilance and passive Pharmacovigilance; • Concept of Various Methods: Spontaneous Reporting, Intensified ADR Reporting, Targeted Reporting, Cohort Event Monitoring, and Electronic Health Record Mining; • Details of Spontaneous Reporting Method of Adverse Drug Reactions; • Details of Cohort Event Monitoring Method in Pharmacovigilance; and • Differences between Spontaneous Reporting and Cohort Event Monitoring.

In simplest way, Pharmacovigilance may be described as the adverse drug events surveillance activity. Based on the surveillance activity the Pharmacovigilance may be divided into: Active Pharmacovigilance and Passive Pharmacovigilance. In Active Pharmacovigilance, active measures are taken to detect the adverse events; and in passive Pharmacovigilance the health professionals and patients are encouraged to volunteer reporting of adverse events.

Active Pharmacovigilance is a prospective surveillance and events are usually detected by active follow up of the patients or their treatment records. It is a systematic approach for more comprehensive data. The Active Pharmacovigilance provides opportunity to obtain denominator of persons exposed to medicines and allowing calculating adverse drug event rates. The methods of Active Pharmacovigilance are: cohort event monitoring, use of registers, record-linkage and screening of laboratory results. Examples of cohort event monitoring: Intensive medicine monitoring programme of New Zealand and prescription event monitoring of England. The Passive Pharmacovigilance relies on spontaneous reporting. The Indian Pharmacovigilance Programme is based on the spontaneous reporting. The spontaneous reporting is the most common method of Pharmacovigilance.

Spontaneous reporting is for the reporting of suspected adverse drug reaction (not events in general) while the cohort event monitoring records all clinical events (not just suspected adverse drug reactions).

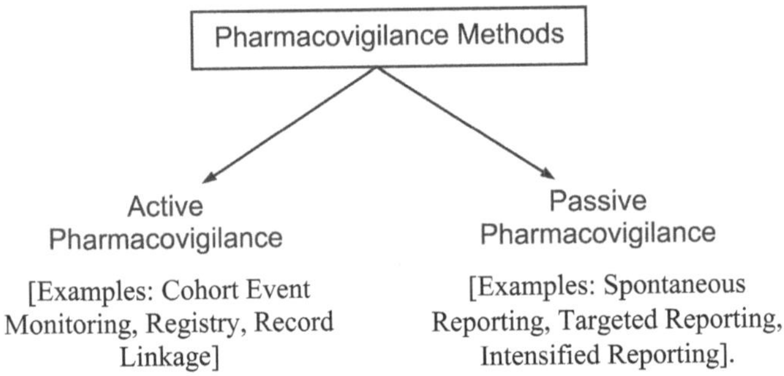

***Cohort Event Monitoring (CEM)*:** Cohort event monitoring is a prospective observational cohort study of adverse events associated with one or more medicines. Cohort means a group of people who share a common characteristic like exposure to a drug within a defined time period. The CEM is basically an observational study during routine clinical practice of a new medicine in the early post-marketing phase and aims at detecting early warning(s).

The salient points of CEM are:

- The study is planned prior to beginning of the treatment with the medication(s);
- All patients who receive the particular medication(s) are made part of the study;
- Every patient is followed up for adverse events since the time of treatment;
- All adverse events are to be recorded and not just the suspected adverse reactions: even minor events, change in pre-existing condition, abnormal change in laboratory tests, lack of effectiveness, admission to hospital including deaths etc.;
- It requires two identical groups of patients receiving different treatment; and

- Sample size: The sample size is determined based on expected adverse event incidence. A cohort of 10 thousand patients gives 95% chance of identifying a specific event with an incidence of 1 in 3000.

The CEM is often inappropriately described as Prescription Event Monitoring [PEM]. The PEM is appropriate when the individual prescription is monitored and the patients receive the medicines based on prescription only. [Patients may also be obtaining medicines without prescriptions].

Example: ADR monitoring of Anti-retroviral medicines. The Government of India launched the ADR monitoring of these medicines under National Pharmacovigilance Programme.

Cohort Event Monitoring	
Pros	**Cons**
Effective in early detection of signals of unsuspected ADRs.	1. Method is more laborious than spontaneous reporting method.
Availability of denominator information allows calculation of incidence rates of ADRs.	2. More expensive method than spontaneous reporting.
Ability to produce a near complete profile of adverse events or adverse drug reactions for the medicines of interest.	3. Being new to health professionals and Pharmacovigilance programme, training is necessary. [Even training is necessary for spontaneous reporting in India as Pharmacovigilance is still in its infancy]
Ability to identify and assess risk and risk factors.	4. Long term follow up may be substantial and needs to be actively managed.
Ability to make accurate comparisons between medicines.	
Ability to establish a pregnancy register and identify problems with pregnancy and common congenital abnormalities.	
Ability to record and examine details of all deaths and provide rates of death.	
Being intensive, the method has the ability to provide clinically significant results rapidly.	
With routine follow up, the method has the ability to detect reduced or failed therapeutic effect. It raises the suspicion of inaccurate diagnosis, poor prescribing, inadequate adherence to treatment, emerging resistance or poor quality medicines.	

Registries: A registry is a record of patients with same characteristics. The registries may be disease specific (disease registry), or specific exposure to drug (drug registry) or type of exposure during a specific life event (pregnancy exposure registry). The registry records the information collected prospectively using standardised questionnaires. This is the most common method used to systematically assess post marketing drug issues in pregnancy. The method is also advocated for assessing the safety of anti-malarial medicines.

Record linkage: Record linkage is the method of assembling information contained in two or more records. The medical or pharmacy or any other relevant record is linked to the safety assessment of medicines. The method is useful for studying long term and late complications by linking well documented complication data and equally documented drug use data at individual level. The method involves data collection through searching of different health database using unique patient identifier. In absence of unique identifying number, any other identifying number like hospital number should be used. The availability of computerised pharmacy or medical records has facilitated the record linkage to safety monitoring programme. The following databases are source of information: register of deaths; register of congenital abnormalities; cancer registers; hospital discharge data; medical and pharmacy billing claims etc.

The quality and extent of drug exposure and diagnostic information is important.

Spontaneous reporting system: Spontaneous adverse drug reaction reporting systems are based on suspected adverse drug reactions. The system collects data about suspected ADRs in a central or regional database. Cases are not collected systematically. A spontaneous report is an unsolicited communication by healthcare professionals or consumers that describes one or more ADRs in a patient who was given one or more medicinal products and that does not derive from a study or any organized data collection scheme. The emphasis is on new findings. The India's National programme does not restrict to only new findings but encourages reporting any reactions that are suspected to be ADR. This helps promoting reporting culture. The terminology 'spontaneous report' is being replaced by individual case safety report.

While different countries or different programmes use different reporting forms, there is need of minimum information for a report to be acceptable. The basic information should be:

- An identifiable source of information / reporter: Name, contact details and status – physician, pharmacist, nurse or patient.
- An identifiable patient: Full name for accurate identification for follow up and to avoid duplication. An identifiable number (if available) and other details like gender, age, weight and height are useful.
- Name(s) of suspected product(s): Brand and Generic Names with dosage form is essential. The dose, mode of administration and indications for use are useful. All other medicines taken at the time of event should also be recorded.
- A description of suspected reaction(s): Date of onset along with a brief clinical description of reaction is essential. Laboratory results (if available), outcome of events (resolved, resolving, no change, death with date etc.) and effect of re-challenge, if any, are useful.

The spontaneous reporting is the most common adverse drug reaction monitoring system and in many countries like India, it is voluntary. Though main limitation of spontaneous reporting systems is their inability to quantify the risk due to non-availability of denominator value, they are the important form of evidence for drug withdrawal or regulatory decisions. Note that all ADRs are not reported; only few are reported.

Examples: Lactic acidosis associated with the biguanides (metformin) was identified.

The form used by National Pharmacovigilance Programme is included in the appendix.

Intensified ADR reporting: This is an extension of spontaneous reporting programme and aims to enhance ADR reporting of specific medicines in early post marketing phase. The procedure is usually followed for new drugs, biological medicines, conditionally approved medicines under exceptional cases, medicines that require additional studies (rare side effects observed during clinical trials). Example: Pharmacovigilance of Antiretroviral medicines under a separate programme.

Targeted spontaneous reporting: This is followed to know more about ADR profile of a specific medicine in the population or to estimate the incidences of a known ADR for a specific medicine in a population. Example: Monitoring renal toxicities related to use of tenofovir based regimen in antiretroviral therapy.

Reasons for inadequate rate of ADR reporting: Dr. Bill Inman described the reasons as seven deadly sins:

1. The mistaken believe that only safe drugs are approved for use.
2. Fear of litigation.
3. A sense of guilt for having caused harm.
4. Ambition to collect and publish a personal series of cases.
5. Ignorance of mechanism for reporting suspected reaction.
6. Diffidence about reporting a mere suspicious.
7. Lethargy or indifference to doctor's responsibility to contribute to the general advancement of knowledge.

Spontaneous Reporting	
Pros	**Cons**
1. Covers the whole population	1. Inherent under reporting – Even in developed countries less than 5% reactions are reported.
2. Includes all medicines	2. Captures only suspected ADRs
3. Continual monitoring throughout the life cycle of a medicine	3. Reporting bias – Seriousness, Severity, Publicity of specific ADRs
4. Details signals of new, rare and serious ADRs can be obtained	4. Difficult to detect – Delayed ADRs
5. Most commonly used Pharmacovigilance method	5. Difficult to calculate reliable rate and measure risk factors
6. Easiest method to establish	6. Deaths are poorly reported
7. Relatively inexpensive compared to CEM	7. Special studies necessary to get accurate information on areas of particular interest – Pregnancy, Paediatrics. The special studies require more funds and thus reduce the cost advantage of spontaneous reporting.
8. Least labour intensive	

Electronic Health Record [EHR] Mining: The electronic health or medical records are rich source of ADR data. They contain detailed patient information and copious longitudinal data. The EHR has emerged as new source that can provide important information which can either complement or improve ADR monitoring programme. The EHR data usually consists of information associated with the process of care and not focusing on adverse drug events. Therefore, ADEs are often sparse in EHR data compared to other types of clinical information: treatments, disorders and symptoms. Besides, the use of EHR for Pharmacovigilance is a new research approach. The signals generated through EHR based different data mining algorithms require further validation. The detailed discussion is beyond the scope of this introductory text.

The comparative characteristics/usefulness of various methods used in Pharmacovigilance are given in the table:

Method	Medicine	Population	Report
Spontaneous Reporting	All medicines – during entire life cycle	All exposed individuals but denominator not known	All suspected ADRs
Intensified Reporting	Specific medicines	All exposed individuals but denominator not known	All suspected ADRs
Targeted Reporting	Specific medicines	Defined Cohort	All suspected ADRs including specific ADRs
CEM	Specific medicines	Defined Cohort	All events
EHR Mining	All medicines	Defined Cohort	All events

Key Messages

- Active Pharmacovigilance refers to the active measures are taken to detect adverse events. Passive Pharmacovigilance refers to spontaneous or voluntary reporting of adverse events.
- Spontaneous reporting is for the reporting of suspected adverse drug reaction (not events in general) while the cohort event monitoring records all clinical events (not just suspected adverse drug reactions).
- Cohort event monitoring, an active Pharmacovigilance programme, compares the incidence of particular adverse event in two identical groups one group taking the medicine of interest while the other group is taking different medicine. It indicates the relative risks.
- All medicines are subject to spontaneous reporting while selected medicines that are to be used widely and are of public health importance are subjected to CEM wherever possible.
- Denominator (number of persons exposed to drug) useful in calculating the risk rate is not known in spontaneous reporting but is known in CEM.
- Spontaneous reporting is the most commonly used method in Pharmacovigilance and India's National Programme follows this method.

Bibliography

1. A Practical Handbook on the Pharmacovigilance of Antiretroviral Medicines, World Health Organization, 2009.
2. Patrick Waller, An introduction to Pharmacovigilance, Wiley –Blackwell, 2010.
3. J. Krska and AR Cox, Adverse drug reactions in Clinical Pharmacy and Therapeutics (Edt by Roger Walker and Cate Whittlesea), Fifth Edition, Churchil Livingstone, Elsevier, 2012.
4. Good Pharmacovigilance Practice Guide, Medicines and Healthcare Products Regulatory Agency, Pharmaceutical Press, 2010.
5. Tanzania Food and Drugs Authority's Pharmacovigilance Training Manual for Healthcare Professionals, Second Edition, 2011.

Chapter 4

Adverse Drug Reactions: Classification, Mechanisms and Susceptibility

"Cured yesterday of my disease, I died last night of my physician/medicine"

After reading this chapter, you should be able to understand and appreciate:
• The types of reactions and their attributes; • The mechanism of such reactions; • Predisposing factors responsible of ADRs.

The main aim of the Pharmacovigilance programme is to identify the unknown adverse reactions of the medicines. The identification of the ADRs is facilitated by understanding their attributes and the classification. The understanding of classification systems help all stake holders of safety monitoring programme developing strategies on avoidance and management of ADRs.

Classification: The Adverse Drug Reactions can be classified in several ways.

Rawlins-Thompson classification: The simplest way of classifying is to divide them into categories: Type A and Type B based on pharmacology: Dose related or non-dose related reactions. This is also called Rawlins-Thompson classification. The type A reactions are related to the known pharmacology of the drug and are dose related. They are reversible on withdrawal of the drug or even simply after dose reduction. The type A reactions are very common accounting about 80% of the total ADRs. In contrast, the type B reactions are qualitatively different from the normal pharmacological action. They are bizarre and cannot be predicted. They cannot be reproduced in animal models too. Thereafter the basic classification is further divided making ADRs into six types: that means four different types – C, D, E and F are added to the system. Type C is dose related and time related, type D is time related and delayed, type E is related to withdrawal reaction and type F is related to unexpected failure of therapy. Type C reactions usually appear during chronic therapy and show a picture less typical for a drug reaction but mimic natural disease. The type D reactions appear long after a treatment or even skipping a generation. Type E reactions can occur after stopping treatment. Type F reactions means failure of efficacy and such reactions are common. The characteristics of each type with examples and management methods are given in the following table.

Type of Adverse Drug Reaction	Attributes	Examples	Management
Type A [Dose Related] / also known as Augmented	• Common [High incidence] • Related to Pharma-cological action [Dose dependent] • Predictable • High Morbidity • Low Mortality • Variable severity but usually mild • Reversible	• Bleeding with warfarin • Hypoglycaemia with sulphonyl-ureas • Headache with glyceryltrinitrate • Bradycardia associated with beta-adrenergic receptor antagonist • Bronchospasm with betablocker use	• Reduction of dose or withholding the drug
Type B [Non-Dose Related] / Also known as Bizarre	• Uncommon [Less incidence] • Unrelated to Pharmacological action [Not dependable on dose] • Unpredictable • Low Morbidity • Variable severity but proportionately more severe than Type A • Irreversible	• Anaphylaxis with penicillin • Hepatitis with halothane • Agranulocytosis with clozapine • Aplastic anaemia caused by chloramphenicol	• Withholding and avoiding in future

Contd...

Type of Adverse Drug Reaction	Attributes	Examples	Management
Type C [Dose Related and Time Related] / Chronic	• Uncommon [Less incidence] • Related to Cumulative dose	• Adrenal suppression with corticosteroids • Osteoporosis with oral steroids	• Reducing the dose or withholding the drug
Type D [Time Related] /Delayed	• Uncommon [Less incidence] • Usually dose related • Appears sometime after use of drug	• Tardive dyskinesia with neuroleptics • Carcinogenesis: DES causing vaginal cancer to next generation members.	Often intractable
Type E [Withdrawal Symptoms]	• Uncommon [Less incidence] • Appears soon after the withdrawal of the drug	• Withdrawal reactions with benzodiazepines • Opiate withdrawal syndrome • Myocardial ischemia after beta-blocker withdrawal	Reintroduction and slow withdrawal of the drug
Type F [Unexpected Failure of Therapy]	• Common (High incidence] • Dose related • Often caused by drug interactions	• Failure of oral contraceptive in presence of enzyme inducer • Resistance to antimicrobials	• Increasing dosage • Provision of concomitant therapy

The above classification is based on the properties of the drug (known pharmacology) and the dose dependence of its effects. It does not take into account some other important factors like: properties of the reactions (the time course of its appearance and severity) and factors accounting for individual variation (genetics, pathological).

> **A drug may cause both type A and type B adverse drug reactions.** Examples - Chlorpromazine [Sedation (A), Cholestatic Jaundice (B)]; Phenytoin [Ataxia (A), Hepatitis (B)] and Warfarin [Bleeding (A), Breast Necrosis (B)]

Though traditionally it is believed that the immunological effects are not dose related but here are some examples that clearly established the dose – response relationship: Hey fever in response to high pollen counts, desensitization by use of increasing dose of cephalosporin. It is, therefore, inappropriate to comment that the type B reactions are not dose dependent.

DoTS system: This three dimensional system was proposed in 2003 by Aroson and Ferner. As the name suggests, the classification is based on three parameters: dose relatedness, time course and susceptibility. The DoTS system classification provides useful means to examine the various factors that describe a reaction and the individual patient's susceptibility.

Dose relatedness: Many adverse drug reactions are related to dose of the drug. In DoTS, the adverse drug reactions are divided into three categories based on dose: toxic effects due to supra-therapeutic dose; collateral effects at standard therapeutic dose; and hyper-susceptibility reactions occurring at sub-therapeutic doses.

Examples: Increased risk of digitalis toxicity with increasing dose [toxic effects]; Osteoporosis due to Corticosteroids [collateral effects]; and Anaphylaxis due to penicillin [hyper-susceptibility reactions].

Time relatedness: The appearance of pharmacological action (including adverse drug reaction) is dependent on concentration of the drug at the site of action and the time at which the drug reaches the site of action.

Examples: Furosemide induces greater diuresis while given as infusion compared to administration as bolus even the dose is same. The toxicity of methotrexate is greater when a low dose is given repeatedly compared to the same amount given as one dose. The reactions can be classified further into time independent reactions and time dependent reactions.

Time independent reactions occur at any time within the treatment period irrespective of duration of treatment. Example: Digoxin toxicity when renal function worsens [Due to change in drug concentration]; and Digoxin toxicity in association with potassium depletion [Action changed without change in concentration].

Time dependent reactions range from rapid and intermediate reactions to delayed reactions. But these terminologies: rapid, immediate and delayed are not clearly defined.

Examples: Rapid reactions [Red man syndrome with vancomycin]; intermediate reactions [Thrombocytopenia due to quinine]; and delayed reactions [Vaginal adenocarcinoma in women who were exposed to diethylstilbestrol in uterus].

Susceptibility: Some persons are more susceptible to adverse reactions than others. The following factors responsible for this susceptibility includes: genetic predisposition, age, gender, altered physiology, disease and drug interaction.

The DoTS system of classification is given in the following table:

Dose relatedness	Time relatedness	Susceptibility
• Toxic effects • Collateral effects • Hyper-susceptibility reactions	• Time independent • Time dependent: • Rapid reactions • Early reactions • Intermediate reactions • Late reactions • Delayed reactions	• Contributing Factors: • Genetic variation • Age • Gender • Altered physiology • Drug interaction • Disease
Example: Anaphylaxis due to penicillin • Dose – Hyper-susceptibility • Time – First dose • Susceptibility – Requires previous sensitization		
Example: Osteoporosis due to corticosteroids • Dose – Collateral effect • Time – Late • Susceptibility – Age and Gender		
Example: Hepatotoxicity due to Isoniazid • Dose – Collateral effect • Time – Intermediate • Susceptibility – Genetic (drug metabolism), age, alcohol, disease		

The DoTS approach has more acceptability as it redresses the issue of some ADRs not fitting into A to F scheme.

It may be appreciated that it may not be possible to classify an ADR into one of the categories discussed above; there may be possibility of expanding or revising the classification further to accommodate the new ADR as identified.

The Adverse Drug Reactions can also be classified on following basis:

The reactions that may occur in any one:

- Drug overdose: Toxic effects associated with over dosing or due to less elimination. Paracetamol hepato-toxicity at high dose (exceeding 4 g daily)
- Drug side effect: Undesirable pharmacologic effects at recommended dose. Anti-histamins cause sedation.
- Drug interaction: Effect of one drug on the effectiveness or toxicity of the other drug. Ferrous sulphate reduces the absorption of tetracycline causing reduced effectiveness of the latter.

Contd...

The reactions that may occur in susceptible individuals:

- Drug intolerance: A low threshold to the normal pharmacological action of a drug.
- Drug idiosyncrasy: A genetically determined, qualitatively abnormal reaction to a drug related to a metabolic or enzyme deficiency.
- Drug allergy: An immunologically mediated reaction, characterised by specificity, transferability by antibodies or lymphocytes, and recurrence on re-exposure.
- Pseudo allergic reaction: A reaction similar to allergic reaction but differs in specificity.

The ADRs at what frequency they affect the people (based on incidence):

- Very Common (incidences in more than 10% exposure),
- Common (incidences in 1% to 10% exposure),
- Uncommon (incidences in 0.1% to 1% exposure),
- Rare (incidences in 0.01% to 0.1% exposure) and
- Very Rare (incidences at less than 0.01% exposure).

Mechanisms of adverse drug reactions: The knowledge of mechanisms of adverse drug reactions helps in avoiding ADRs during medicine use. While it is difficult to categorise the mechanisms into discrete categories, they may be grouped into the following main types:

1. Pharmacological (Physiological) effects.
2. Drug – Drug Interactions.
3. Triggering an immunological action.

The genetic variation and pathological conditions too influence the occurrence of ADRs.

Pharmacological (Physiological) effects: Examples – Non-steroidal anti-inflammatory drugs or corticosteroids may cause gastric haemorrhage or peptic ulcer. Aspirin, an anti-inflammatory agent, may cause bleeding due to its anti-platelet effect. Barbiturates are sedatives but can cause respiratory depression. Antihistamins have sedation as adverse effects.

The drug may cause its effects at another site (which is not desired). Glyceryl trinitrate (used in angina) may cause headache.

The individual's ability to process the drug (including the formulation design) and the pharmacokinetic parameters are also responsible for ADRs. A change in drug formulation may affect the bioavailability. A change in formulation in phenytoin capsule (calcium sulphate is replaced by lactose as diluent) was responsible for causing neurological disorders in 1960s due to increased phenytoin concentration in blood. Impairment in drug metabolism or drug elimination may lead to accumulation of drug in the body causing toxicity.

Drug – Drug interactions: Patients on polypharmacy are more likely to have ADRs. All the three types of drug interactions – pharmaceutical, pharmacodynamic and pharmacokinetic interaction may cause ADRs (may increase toxicity or reduce therapeutic efficacy). An Angiotensin Converting Enzyme (ACE) inhibitor and a potassium sparing diuretic, if given together, may result in hyperkalaemia and cardiac arrhythmias. Cimetidine inhibits the metabolism of warfarin and thereby increases the latter's anti-coagulant effect leading to bleeding.

Triggering an immunological action: This leads to allergic or hypersensitivity reactions. These types of reactions do not resemble pharmacological actions. Drug either alone or in combination with antigenic proteins precipitates allergic reactions. The severity of allergic reaction, in general, related to the route of administration. Anaphylactic shocks are more common with injections. Injection of penicillin may cause anaphylaxis. Hence, penicillin allergy is always tested before giving the full dose. Many drugs cause skin allergy like pruritis. Some may cause fatal Stevens – Johnson Syndrome.

Susceptibility to adverse drug reactions: Some people are more susceptible than others to ADRs due to presence of risk factors. The knowledge of the risk factors provides an opportunity for avoiding or minimizing the number of adverse effects and also reducing the harm to the patients. The risk factors that are responsible for susceptibility to ADRs can be grouped into three categories: factors associated with the patient; factors associated with the medicine; and factors associated with the environment.

Risk factors associated with the patient

- **Age:** The elderly and neonates are at greatest risk. The elderly persons, with age related decline in metabolism and elimination coupled with co-morbid conditions, are more susceptible to ADRs. A decreased volume of distribution and decreased rate of elimination result in increased drug concentration which in turn increases the probability of adverse drug effects.

  Example: All central nervous system depressants are liable to have greater effect than normal leading to confusion. Barbiturates may lead to immobility. Flucloxacillin induced jaundice and hepatitis is more common in elderly persons.

Children differ from adults in terms of body composition; and the ability to metabolize and eliminate. The immature blood – brain barrier makes the children more sensitive to morphine. Example – Aspirin is associated with Reye's syndrome in children.

- ***Size, weight and height or body mass index:*** The normal doses are designed based on average adult body weight of 70 kg. Such dose may result in higher drug concentration in those of lower body weight leading to drug toxicity.
- ***Genetic polymorphism:*** Patients' genetic makeup makes them more susceptible to ADRs.

  Example: Stevens-Johnson Syndrome and Toxic Epidermal Necrolysis are associated with carbamazepine and phenytoin and more common in population of China, Thailand, Malaysia, Indonesia, the Philippines and Taiwan than people of India and Japan. The readers are advised to read the chapter on Pharmacogenetics.
- ***Gender (pregnancy):*** Women are generally at higher risk.

  Examples: Thalidomide's association with birth defects. The psychiatric adverse events with mefloquine are more common in females.
- ***Co-morbidities:*** The co-morbidities such as congestive cardiac failure, respiratory disorders, diabetes, hepatic, renal impairment etc., have profound influence on drug action. The respiration depressant drugs [opiates, barbiturates] may precipitate respiratory failure in patients with a malfunctioning respiratory centre [raised intracranial pressure]. The patients with raised intracranial pressure may be restless. The respiratory depressant, if used for quietening the restlessness, may cause respiratory failure.

  Digitalis causes cardiac arrhythmia in patients with myocardial infarction.
- ***Renal or Liver damage:*** Reduction in hepatic and renal function substantially increases the risk of ADRs.

Risk factors associated with medicine

- ***Dose:*** Higher the dose more is the risk. Paracetamol exceeding daily dose of 4 g increases the risk of liver toxicity.
- ***Duration of therapy:*** Benzodiazepine dependence occurs when treatment last several months or years. When the drug is suddenly stopped withdrawal symptoms appear.

- ***Previous exposure:*** Hypersensitivity to penicillin occurs due to prior exposure.
- ***Polypharmacy:*** The use of multiple medicines simultaneously increases the chances of potential interaction.

Risk associated with environment

- ***Tobacco use:*** Smoking increases the enzyme activity in the liver. Smoking increases the removal of theophyline requiring dose adjustment. Smoking decreases the absorption of insulin leading to delayed action. Smokers do require higher dose of glibenclamide.
- ***Alcohol or other drugs:*** Alcohol increases the risk of liver toxicity of paracetamol. There is increased risk of gastric irritation and bleeding with aspirin when taken together with alcohol.
- ***Diet:*** Grape fruit juice is an enzyme inhibitor. When taken with calcium channel blocker, the grape fruit increases the plasma concentration leading to adverse effects.
- ***Medicines of other system:*** A herbal medicine, St. John's Wort, is an enzyme inducer and reduces the effectiveness of ciclosporin.

Key Messages

- The ADRs can be classified at least in two basic ways:
  - Rawlins – Thompson Method: Type A, B, C, D, E and F. Type A is related to pharmacologic action and is dose dependent. Type B not related to pharmacology of the drug and is dose independent.
  - DoTS System: Dose relatedness, Time relatedness and Susceptibility.
- The mechanisms for ADRs: Pharmacological effects, Drug-Drug interactions and Triggering an immunologic action.
- The risks factors that make a person more vulnerable to ADRs are:
  - Patient related factors – age, weight, body mass index, genetic polymorphism, gender, co-morbidities, renal and liver damage;
  - Medicine related factors – dose, duration, previous exposure, and polypharmacy;
  - Environment related factors – tobacco use, alcohol intake, diet and medicine of other system.

Bibliography

1. Roger Walker and Cate Whittlesea (Editors), Clinical Pharmacy and Therapeutics, 5th Edition, Churchil Livingston, Elsevier, 2012.
2. J K Aronson and R E Ferner, Joining the DoTS: new approach to classifying adverse drug reactions, British Medical Journal, Nov 22, 2003.
3. Patrick Waller, An Introduction to Pharmacovigilance, Wiley – Blackwell, UK, 2010.
4. Ronald D. Mann and Elizabeth Andrews (Ed), Pharmacovigilance, Second Edition, John Wiley & Sons Limited, England, 2007.

Chapter 5

Assessment of Adverse Events' Reports

"I firmly believe that if the whole of the material medica, as now used, could be sunk to the bottom of the sea, it would be all better for mankind and the all the worse for the fishes".

Oliver Wendell Holmes

After reading this chapter, you should be able to understand and appreciate:
• Methods of severity assessment of suspected ADR. • Methods of causality assessment of suspected ADR. • Methods of preventability assessment of suspected ADR and strategies available to prevent ADRs in health facilities.

The functions of any Pharmacovigilance programme includes monitoring, detecting, reporting, evaluating, and documenting medicine safety data and providing feedback to the reporters, health professionals and the drug regulators. Once the information is collected they need to be analysed to determine the adverse events severity, probable causality and preventability.

Severity: The severity of adverse drug reaction may be classified as:

- *Severe*: Example – Reaction is fatal or life threatening;
- *Moderate*: Example – Reaction requires antidote, medical procedure, or hospitalization;
- *Mild*: Example – the symptoms require only the discontinuation of the drug therapy; and
- *Incidental*: Example – There are very mild symptoms where the patients can choose whether to continue medicine or discontinue.

The severity assessment is best done using modified Hartwig and Siegel scale. The details are given in the tabular form:

Category	Level	Characteristics
Mild	Level - 1	• The ADR requires no change in the treatment with the suspected drug. OR
	Level - 2	• The ADR requires that the suspected drug be withheld, discontinued, or otherwise changed. • No antidote or other treatment is required. • There is no increase in length of hospital stay.
Moderate	Level – 3	• The ADR requires that the suspected drug be withheld, discontinued, or otherwise changed. • An antidote or other treatment is required. • There is no increase in length of stay, OR
	Level – 4	• (a) Any level-3 ADR that increases the length of stay at least by one day. OR
		• (b) The ADR is the cause of admission.
Severe	Level - 5	• Any level- 4 ADR that requires intensive medical care. OR
	Level – 6	• The ADR causes permanent harm to the patient. OR
	Level - 7	• The ADR either directly or indirectly leads to the death of the patient.

Causality: After identifying a suspected ADR, it is important to demonstrate a causal relationship between the drug and the untoward clinical event. Establishing causality is a process which begins by examining the relationship between the drug and the event. Causality assessment is used to determine the likelihood that a drug caused a suspected ADR. There are a number of methods used to judge causation with each one having its own merits and demerits. The methods require some level of expert judgement to apply.

'World Health Organisation' and the 'Naranjo Probability' Scale are simple to apply. They are generally accepted and most widely used methods for causality assessment in clinical practice. These two methods offer objective, reliable and valid causality assessment of ADRs along with the convenience of being easy to apply methods.

WHO causality categories: There are six standardised causality categories designed by WHO: certain (or definite), probable, possible, unlikely, unclassified (or conditional), and un-assessable (or unclassifiable). With the permission of World Health Organization, the characteristics requirements for each causality category are reproduced from *A Practical Handbook on the Pharmacovigilance of Antiretroviral Medicines, 2009*:

Category	Requirements for inclusion in a specific category
Certain (or, definite)	1. The event is a specific clinical or laboratory phenomenon. 2. The time elapsed between the administration of the drug and the occurrence of the event is plausible. [Requirements: dates of drug administration and the date of onset of the event must be known] 3. The event cannot be explained by concomitant disease or any other drug or chemical. [Requirement: Details of other medicines taken must be known. The report must also state if there were no other medicines in use. If this is unknown, then doubt exists and the event cannot be included in this category). 4. The patient recovered within a plausible length of time following withdrawal of the drug. [The date of withdrawal of the drug and the time taken for recovery should be known. If these dates are unknown, then doubt exists and the event cannot be included in this category.] 5. The same event recurred following re-challenge with the same drug alone. [Requirement: The report must state the outcome of re-challenge. If this is unknown, then doubt exists and the event cannot be included in this category.] *It cannot be classified as Certain if there has been no re-challenge, or the outcome of the re-challenge is unknown.*
Probable	1. The event is a specific clinical or laboratory phenomenon. 2. The time elapsed between the administration of the drug and the occurrence of the event is plausible. [The dates of drug administration and the date of onset of the event must be known.] 3. The event cannot be explained by concurrent disease or any other drug or chemical. [The details of other medicines taken must be known. The report must also state if there were no other medicines in use. If this is unknown, then doubt exists and the event cannot be included in this category.] 4. The patient recovered within a plausible length of time following withdrawal of the drug. [The date of drug withdrawal and the time taken for recovery should be known.] 5. Re-challenge did not occur, or the result is unknown. *It cannot be classified as Probable if there has been no de-challenge or the result of de-challenge is not known or the outcome of the event is unknown or if there are other possible causes of the event.*

Contd...

Category	Requirements for inclusion in a specific category
Possible	1. The time elapsed between the administration of the drug and the occurrence of the event is plausible. [The date of administration and the date of onset of the event must be known.] 2. The outcome of withdrawal of the suspect medicine is not known, and/or medicine might have been continued and the final outcome is not known; and/or 3. There might be no information on withdrawal of medicine; and /or 4. The event could be explained by concomitant disease or use of other drugs or chemicals; and / or 5. There might be no information on the presence or absence of other medicines. 6. Deaths cannot be coded as probable because there is no opportunity to see the effect of the withdrawal of the drug. If there is a plausible time relationship, a death should be coded as possible. 7. In addition to deaths, there is a further group of events that do not fit the relationship assessment process and the coding can vary. Consider the following examples: • Myocardial infarction: Many patients recover from this event as part of the natural history of the disease and, with very few exceptions, recovery is not a response to withdrawal of a drug. Hence the result of 'de-challenge' is meaningless. This type of reaction may be coded as 'possible'. • Stroke: Some patients recover fully, some partially, some remain severely disabled and some die. All these outcomes are part of the natural history of the disease and, with very few exceptions, are unrelated to drug withdrawal. Again, the result of 'de-challenge' is usually meaningless. This type of reaction may be coded as 'Possible'. • Acute anaphylaxis immediately following an injection: Here there is an obvious direct relationship, but the usual parameters for establishing relationship, e.g., de-challenge do not apply. In this example, best category for relationship is 'certain'.
Unlikely	1. The event occurred with a duration to onset that makes a causal effect improbable with the drug being considered. [The pharmacology of the drug and the nature of the event should be considered in arriving at this conclusion]; and /or

Contd...

Category	Requirements for inclusion in a specific category
	2. The event commenced before the first administration of the drug; and/ or 3. The drug was withdrawn and this made no difference to the event when clinically recovery would be expected. [This would not apply for some serious events such as myocardial infarction, or events causing permanent damage]; and / or It is strongly suggestive of a non-causal relationship if the drug was continued and the event resolved.
Unclassified (or, Conditional)	These are reports with insufficient data to establish a relationship and more data are expected. This is a temporary repository and the category for these events will be finalized when the new data become available.
Un-assessable	1. An event has occurred in association with a drug, but there are insufficient data to make an assessment. 2. Some of the data may be contradictory or inconsistent. 3. Details of the report cannot be supplemented or verified.

The WHO causality system is basically a combined assessment, taking into account the clinical-pharmacological aspects of the case history and the quality of documentation of observation, while prior knowledge of the ADR plays a less significant part.

Alert on WHO Causality Assessment:

- When there is no re-challenge or the outcome of re-challenge is unknown: Relationship cannot be termed CERTAIN.
- When there is no de-challenge or the outcome of de-challenge is unknown: Relationship cannot be termed PROBABLE.
- When the outcome of the event is unknown: relationship can be termed PROBABLE.
- When there are other possible causes of the event: relationship cannot be termed PROBABLE.

Naranjo probability scale (Algorithm): The Naranjo Probability Scale is another widely used scale for causality assessment. This uses questionnaires and points are added or taken away based on the response to each question. The total score is then used to decide the category as: definite, probable, possible or doubtful. It is helpful for assessing unexpected ADRs and useful for evaluators with little experience.

Questions	Yes	No	Don't Know	Categorization
1. Are there previous conclusive reports on this reaction?	+1	0	0	If the total score is more than 9, then certain; if the total score is between 5 – 8, then probable; if the total score is between 1 – 4, then possible and if the total score is 0 (zero), then unlikely.
2. Did the ADR appear after the suspected drug was administered?	+2	-1	0	
3. Did the ADR improve when the drug was discontinued or specific antagonist was administered?	+1	0	0	
4. Did the ADR reappear with re-challenge (administered again)?	+2	-1	0	
5. Are there alternative causes for the ADR (other than the drug) that could solely have caused the reaction?	-1	+2	0	
6. Did the reaction appear when placebo was given?	-1	+1	0	
7. Was the drug detected in blood (or other fluids) at toxic levels?	+1	0	0	
8. Was the reaction more severe when the dose was increased, or less severe when the dose was decreased?	+1	0	0	
9. Did the patient have a similar reaction to the same or similar drug in any previous exposure?	+1	0	0	
10. Was the ADR confirmed by any objective evidence?	+1	0	0	

Points to remember:

- The quality of data and documentation influence the reliability of the method. Often, individual systems of causality assessment are non-comparable.
- The relationship of a single report can be established but firm opinion may not be possible.
- A causality assessment is viewed as provisional and subject to change when new information or knowledge is made available.
- It is often unethical to re-challenge with the patients like who experience severe haematological toxicities. Thus without a re-challenge, it is difficult to achieve causality rating of 'definite'.

Preventability: Preventing Adverse Drug Reactions are not only possible but are necessary in both patient's and health system's interest. It has been reported that more than 50% adverse drug reactions may be preventable. Most ADRs are related to the prescribing of an incorrect dose or the administration of a drug to the patient with a known allergy.

There are several instruments/scales suggested for assessing the preventability of an ADR and they vary widely. However, they share the same basis for defining preventability. It seems Modified Schumock and Thornton scale is more acceptable. This scale divides preventability into three categories as: definitely preventable, probably preventable and not preventable.

Definitely Preventable	Parameters to be assessed	Comment
	1. Was there a history of allergy or previous reaction to the drug?	Answering YES to one or more of the parameters implies that ADR is definitely preventable. (If the answers are all NEGATIVE, proceed to next section given below)
	2. Was the drug involved inappropriate for the patient's clinical condition?	
	3. Was the dose, route or frequency of administration inappropriate for the patient's age, weight or disease state?	
Probably Preventable	1. Was the required therapeutic drug monitoring or other necessary laboratory tests not performed?	Answering YES to one or more of these parameters implies that ADR is probably preventable. [if answer are all NEGATIVE to these parameters, proceed to next section below]
	2. Was a documented drug interaction involved in the ADR?	
	3. Was poor compliance involved in the ADR?	
	4. Was a preventable measure not administered to the patient?	
	5. If a preventable measure was administered, was it inadequate or inappropriate? ANSWER NO IF THIS QUESTION IS NOT APPLICABLE.	
Not Preventable	If the ADR does not fall into the above two categories: definitely preventable or probably preventable.	

Preventing ADRs in Health Facilities Level: The following actions are advocated at health facility level to promote medicines' safety and help reducing occurrence of ADRs:

- Documenting the previous history of ADR of the patient.
- Introducing ADR reporting programme and encourage healthcare professionals to participate.
- Educating and sensitizing staff on need of ADRs through continuing professional development programme, through drug bulletins, and through reports of collected adverse events.
- Closely monitoring the high risk medicines.
- Closely monitoring high risk patients like pregnant women, breast feeding women, elderly persons, and persons with kidney or liver impairment.
- Reviewing the adverse reaction report on regular basis and updating the healthcare staff on incidence and impact of ADRs.
- Revise the medicine list and treatment guidelines in the light of significant ADRs.

Key Messages

- The adverse event reports are required to be evaluated for severity, probable causality and preventability.
- The severity of adverse drug reaction is classified as severe, moderate, mild and incidental.
- WHO scale and Naranjo probability scale are two widely accepted methods of causality assessment. WHO has six causality categories: certain (definite), probable, possible, unlikely, unclassified (or, conditional) and un-assessable (un-classifiable).
- Naranjo probability scale is based on the scoring system for a set of 10 questions: Score more than 9 means certain, score between 5 to 8 means probable, score between 1 to 4 means possible, and score 0 means unlikely.
- Modified Schumock and Thornton scale is an acceptable method for classifying preventability of adverse drug events: definitely preventable, probably preventable and not preventable.

Bibliography

1. Kathleen Holloway and Terry Green, Drug and Therapeutics Committees, A Practical Guide, World Health Organization and Management Sciences for Health, 2003.

2. A Practical Handbook on the Pharmacovigilance of Antiretroviral Medicines, World Health Organization, 2009.
3. K. G. Revikumar and B. D. Miglani, A Textbook of Pharmacy Practice, First Edition, Career Publications, 2009.
4. SK Gupta (Ed), Textbook of Pharmacovigilance, First Edition, Jaypee Brothers Medical Publishers (P) Ltd., 2011.
5. Ron Mann and Elizabeth Andrews (Ed), Pharmacovigilance, Second Edition, John Wiley & Sons Ltd, 2007.

Chapter 6

Signal: Identification and Strengthening

"I do not want two diseases: one nature made and one doctor made".

Napoleon Bonaparte

After reading this chapter, you should be able to understand and appreciate:
• Definition of Signal. • Methods of Signal Identification. • Evaluation of Signals (signal strengthening). • WHO leadership in Signal Detection.

During clinical trials with limited time and limited exposure, all adverse effects are not identified. As some of the ADRs can be identified only after long exposure of the drug and to large population, the safety monitoring of the product continues after marketing approval. The primary objective of the safety monitoring of the medicine (also known as Pharmacovigilance) is the early detection of previously unknown adverse effects of the medicines. The early detection of the safety issues would help promoting safe use of medicines. The early warning sign is known as signal. Similarly in risk management process, identification of the possible hazard is the first step. After identifying the hazard, it is investigated further and if required, action is initiated to minimise the risk.

It is necessary to provide right environment for health professionals to be observant and critical in their diagnoses and therapy, so that they do not miss any piece of new information that may make therapy safer. The careful, informed, routine, systematic and standardised clinical review of reports of adverse drug events with the recording and appropriate collation of good data provides the quickest and justified way of identifying the previously unsuspected adverse reactions. It is important that safety of all medicines is monitored throughout their marketed life.

The World Health Organization defines Signal as "Reported information on a possible causal relationship between an adverse event and a drug, the relationship being unknown or incompletely documented previously."

The important points to remember are:

- The new information relevant to drug safety may come from different sources: reports of adverse events, clinical or non-clinical experiments, and published articles.
- Safety signal is suggestive of something new which would be worth further investigating. It is not confirmed safety issue.
- Newness may be on emerging trends and changes on specificity, severity, and/or rate of occurrence of a previously known adverse drug reaction. It may not be fully new.
- Safety signal precedes further investigation in determining whether or not a possible association rises to the level of warranting further action.

The continuing safety monitoring system should be available to: ensure regular screening of all sources of information to identify any potential signal; ensure appropriate action in response to new evidence that impacts on the known risk-benefit ratio; and communicate appropriately on risk-benefit changes to the drug regulating authority, healthcare professionals and the patients.

The following criteria are indicators for identifying events for investigation: good data; the event is clinically relevant; several reports showing credible and strong relationship with the drug (certain or probable); and the event would be significant if validated.

Spontaneous reporting of Adverse Events is the most common method used in Pharmacovigilance. It is helpful in detecting type B effects such as allergic or idiosyncratic reactions. The type B reactions occur only in minority of patients and usually unrelated to dosage and they are serious, unexplained and unpredictable too. Spontaneous reporting is also helpful in detecting unusual type A effects. The type A effects are pharmacologic effects of the drug and are dose related. Other sources of signal are: prescription event monitoring, large automated data resources on morbidity and drug use, case control surveillance and follow up studies. Type C effects (these effects related to an increased frequency of spontaneous disease) are difficult to study.

Methods of Signal Identification

I. ***Clinical assessment of individual events*:**

Careful, routine, standardised clinical assessment of individual reports with alertness to the possibility of a signal is the quickest method of detecting signal. The following points provide a guide to be adopted sequentially:

- When it is sensed to be a new type of adverse reaction, a search for records of similar events is warranted to confirm the opinion;
- The database needs to be checked for similar reports or clinically related terms;
- The adverse reaction should be checked in the reference source/s;
- If there is no reference of the occurrence of the event, investigation is needed to be continued.

A single report of a suspected adverse reaction can only rarely be considered as a signal itself. One can never be certain about a causal relationship between drug exposure and the adverse event on the basis of one individual case. It is only through on-going analysis of the collection of events that a potential signal is generated.

II. ***Systematic review of multiple case reports*:** All the events in the database for the drug(s) of interest are to be reviewed at regular intervals. The periodicity of the systemic review of cumulative data for the purpose of signal detection depends on the amount of safety data received or available in the database. One month frequency may be acceptable.

There are various methods for review of data as a part of signal detection, ranging from manual review of individual cases to the use of computer algorithms of drug safety database (also known as data mining). Every method has its own advantages and disadvantages. Individual case review allows complete evaluation of every aspect of the case but often is an issue of resource constraint. Simple counts of number of suspected adverse reactions or a frequency analysis can highlight the appearance of a new reaction or an increase in the occurrence of a known reaction. It is necessary to consider at what point an increase in number or frequency of a suspected adverse reaction becomes significant. Is the increase due to increase in sales?

III. *Record linkage*:

Literally the record linkage is the systematic bringing together of the records of the individuals in a large population. In Pharmacovigilance, record linkage is the linkage of patient specific information that is stored separately.

The record linkage is possible on the availability of a unique identifier for the patients either in the health system or in hospital record. This same identifier must be recorded with the patient details in the cohort database. The process involves matching the details in cohort database with that of hospital or other records. This would enable to see the details of the patient: whether the patient died and the cause of death; whether patient was admitted to hospital and the diagnosis etc. The review result is recorded in the patient's database in cohort.

An unexpectedly high rate of a particular event like liver damage may represent a signal.

IV. *Automated signal detection*:

The automated statistical methods used in the analysis of safety data include the proportional reporting ratio (PRR). PRR is a method that uses software to measure the proportion of reports in the database with a particular drug – event combination and compares this proportion with that for the same event in the reports for all other drugs combined. This requires a large set of data and exceptionally high reporting of suspected adverse reaction of one type or in one system organ class. If the PRR for a particular drug –event combination is significantly high, and it is not a recognised reaction, it may represent a signal. PRR methods are somewhat experimental and they lack reliability.

Though earlier PRR system was used by both pharmaceutical companies and the regulatory authorities, the system is being replaced by empirical Bayesian methods. While it is beyond the scope of this text giving more details of Bayesian methods, a brief description is given. The commonly used Bayesian methods include: The Bayesian Confidence Propagation Neural Network (BCPNN) and Multi – Item Gamma Poisson Shrinker (MGPS), for the purpose of signal detection. Medicines and Healthcare Products Regulatory Agency (MHRA) of UK employs MGPS and Uppsala Monitoring

Centre (UMC) uses BCPNN (and data mining) techniques for signal detection.

All signals identified from statistical programmes require subsequent clinical evaluation.

V. ***Other sources of information*:**

The responsible professional should look into the periodic safety update reports, information from new non-clinical research, post marketing studies, clinical trials and from other initiatives such as surveys and registries. The few good sources too can be explored for information on ADRs: Martindale's The Complete Drug Reference, The Physician's Desk Reference, and Micromedex online drug reference etc.

If there is no good evidence of an event being recognised as an adverse reaction in two – or more of these references and if warranted clinically, it should be investigated further as a possible signal.

Signal Detection Algorithms (SDAs): They have been accepted as the vital tools used with reasonable predictive accuracy in signalling adverse events. For identifying safety signals of adverse events from spontaneous reports, data mining techniques are increasingly used to supplement the traditional expert review of reports and to analyse the large volume of accumulated data more rapidly. These data mining techniques are known as SDAs.

The SDAs are the tools used to analyse the databases of spontaneous reports for concealed associations between drugs and reported adverse events that may evade the scrutiny of manual assessment. SDAs are designed to compute surrogate measures of statistical association between drug-event pairs reported in a database. These measures are often interpreted as signal scores, with larger values representing stronger associations indicating more likely to represent true ADRs. The regulatory bodies like USFDA regularly uses SDAs to the Adverse Events Reports in order to monitor, prioritise, and identify new safety signals of Adverse Drug Events that require further investigation.

***Signal strengthening*:** The potential signals generally require further investigation for making a decision whether the product in question caused the event. It is necessary to perform a review of the case(s) that prompted the initial signal alert in addition to performing a search for any additional cases and other information relevant to the issue. The clinical evaluation of identified signals is called strengthening of signals. The indepth review of the cases is usually based on the following principles:

(i) Reviewing other experience: Look for the all available data source for similar reports. While performing searches, the search terms are carefully selected to ensure all relevant cases are retrieved;

(ii) Searching for non-random patterns: Examination of data on a group of reports may show patterns that are not random, and in the absence of biases, non-random pattern suggest that the event may be related to the medicine. Example – when compared with the cohort, if the rate of events in women and men are significantly different, then drug effect could be one of the reasons;

(iii) Reviewing the pharmacology: To find out whether there is any plausible mechanism by which the medicine could cause the event;

(iv) Consulting expert safety review panel and other experts – The reviewers are asked to review the case reports using their clinical experience and pharmacological knowledge

(v) Undertaking epidemiological studies: The following studies may be essential: cohort studies, case control studies, record linkage studies, and population database studies;

(vi) Communicating to stakeholders: Effective and well presented communication of the signal to all stakeholders seeking their feedback would help validating the signal. The following stakeholders may be considered seeking their opinion: expert safety review panel, regulatory authority, health professionals, pharmaceutical company, Uppsala Monitoring ADR bulletin and medical journals.

World Health Organization's Leadership in Signal Detection: WHO programme for International Drug Monitoring is managed by its collaborating centre, the Uppsala Drug Monitoring Centre. The UMC team regularly searches Vigibase for new signals and communicates the results to the regulatory authorities of member countries. Vigibase is the name for the WHO International ADR database. UMC uses Bayesian Confidence Propagation Neural Network [BCPNN] technique for finding new drug-ADR combinations likely to be signals through quantitative filtering of the data. This focuses clinical review on the potentially most important combinations of drugs and adverse drug reactions. Other useful information can also be obtained from Vigibase such as variation in ADR patterns in different countries. The causes of such differences may be due to different ingredients in the formulation, different dosage or different indications for use.

Contd...

The Review Process: The data in Vigibase is scanned using automated data mining programme, the BCPNN, to produce a database with case information and occurrence of drug – ADRs including a content table. The results are presented in a computerised table called **Combination Database.** At this stage the list is neither filtered nor analyzed or reviewed. The list is sent periodically to the National centres who review its international contents for issue of relevance to their own country.

Based on statistical threshold and the Information Component (IC) values the promising drug-ADR pairs are copied into **Association Database**. They are considered worth examining further. The IC values for drug – event combinations can be plotted as graphs over time to examine any trend. A positive signal will have IC values that become more significant over time as more cases are included.

A filtering process is applied to narrow down the number of combinations for review and to focus on the areas of the greatest importance. This is to establish a priority focus through predefined algorithms which may also consider: rapid reporting increase, serious reaction and new drug, special interest reactions, to give a manageable number of combinations.

Then the prioritised drug – ADR combinations are checked for their occurrence in the available literatures such Martindale's Complete Drug Reference, Physician's Drug Reference, Drug Dex etc., to see what is known and whether the combinations have merits to pass to reviewers for indepth study. For drugs where the reaction is not available in the literature or not fully described, it is necessary to retrieve the complete case reports from Vigibase. These are then sent to appropriate expert in the review panel with a request to assess the evidence for the relationship of the reaction to the suspected drug. The material for review is divided into System Organ Classes (SOC) for the ADRs and Anatomical, Therapeutic, Chemical (ATC) Groups for the drugs.

The International experts drawn from different countries are requested to assess the case reports using their clinical experience and pharmacological knowledge. Analysis of potential signals includes checking the available case data and making literature searches. After assessing the cases, including the judgement on the causal strength of the drug –ADR association, the reviewer drafts a short report on the signal if felt worth notifying to the National centres. After review within the UMC, the text of the report is included in SIGNAL for distribution to National Centres. SIGNAL is the restricted publication of UMC.

Contd...

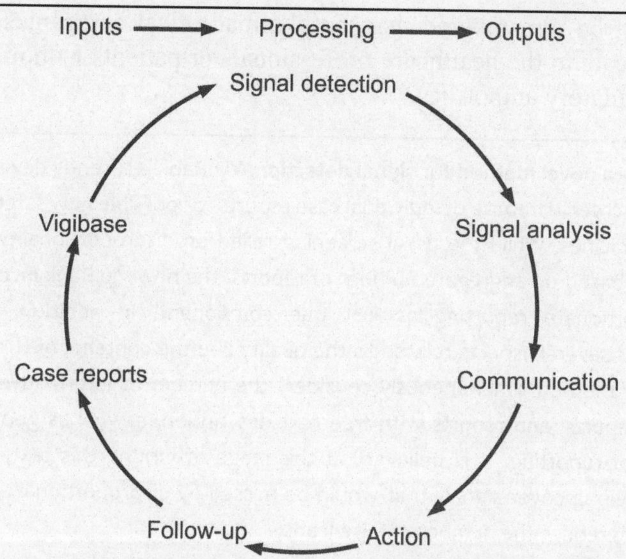

Source: View Point, Part 2, the Uppsala Monitoring Centre, 2004.

Fig. 6.1: Flow Chart Showing the Principal Elements of the Pharmacovigilance at the International Level [From Report to Final]

While it is not possible to have equally effective Pharmacovigilance programme in every country, WHO's International database provides enough information on safety issues to the regulatory authorities and pharmaceutical companies, of resource constrained countries, to take appropriate action reducing medicine use related harms.
[Source: View Point – Part 2, *the* Uppsala Monitoring Centre, 2004.]

Investigation of signals is an iterative process and at each stage there should be consideration of the need for communication with regulatory authorities and /or implementation of risk minimisation measures. When a new signal is identified, it is important to consider the potential of increased risk and change in its risk – benefit. The pharmaceutical companies should notify the regulatory authority immediately of any change in the balance of risks and benefits of their products. Upon confirmation of new signal for a product, the following action may be initiated:

- Variation of the summary of product characteristics or product information leaflets;
- Provision of safety information directly to healthcare professionals and public.

It must be remembered that the pharmaceutical companies must not communicate to the healthcare professionals or patients without approval of the regulatory authorities.

VigiRank- a novel method for signal detection: VigiRank is recently developed by UMC to screen database of individual case reports for possible new safety signals with medicines. While the usual screening relied on disproportionality analysis which is based on aggregate number of reports, the new VigiRank incorporates disproportionate reporting as just one component. In addition, VigiRank considers several aspects related to the quality and the contents of the reports. The new method simultaneously considers the number of informative reports, recent reports, and reports with free text description, as well as geographical spread of reporting. It is believed, at this stage of writing this text, VigiRank would help uncover signals that would be missed by disproportionality analysis alone and reduce the number of false leads.

[Uppsala Reports October 2014]

Key Messages

- One of the most important aspects of drug – safety monitoring of marketed products is the identification and analysis of new, medically important findings that might influence the use of medicines.
- Serious signals that appear to be new and relate to new drugs usually elicit regulatory action. Less serious signals though have significant morbidity or compliance, may not be investigated so vigorously even when the numbers build up.
- The factors that determine the evidence contained in a signal: quantitative strength of association, consistency of the data, exposure response relationship, biological plausibility, experimental findings, possible analysis, and the nature and quality of data.
- The BCPNN runs on all reported events worldwide and therefore, there are greater chances of finding more reports of the suspect drug – event combination.
- The WHO programme usually considers signals if they are involved in more than one country.

Bibliography

1. Ronald HB Meyboom *et al*, Principles of Signal Detection in Pharmacovigilance, Drug Safety, 16(6), June 1997.
2. Guideline on Good Pharmacovigilance Practices, Module IX-Signal Management, European Medicines Agency, 22 June 2012.
3. Atsuko Shibata and Manfred Hauben, Pharmacovigilance, Signal Detection and Signal Intelligence Review, 14th International Conference on Information Fusion, Chicago, USA, 2011.
4. Patrick Waller, An introduction to Pharmacovigilance, Wiley –Blackwell, 2010.
5. A Practical Handbook on the Pharmacovigilance of Antiretroviral Medicines, World Health Organization, 2009.

Chapter 7

Quality Assurance in Pharmacovigilance

"Fortunately a surgeon who uses the wrong side of the scalpel cuts his own fingers and not the patient's; if the same applied to drugs, they would have investigated very carefully a long time ago".

Rudolph Bucheim
Beitrage Zur Arzneimitteellehre **(1849)**

After reading this chapter, you should be able to understand and appreciate:
• Concept of quality assurance and quality control in Pharmacovigilance system; • Concept of Good Pharmacovigilance; • Quality Assurance Process in Pharmacovigilance; and • Indicators which may be used to assess a pharmacovigilance system.

In a quality conscious world, the pharmacovigilance system needs to ensure that the key activities and processes are being performed in accordance with expected procedures promoting good pharmacovigilance practice. There are two main stakeholders: National Medicine Regulatory Authority and Marketing Authorization Holders who are responsible for ensuring the functioning of quality system in pharmacovigilance activities.

The quality management system aims to build the quality to the product or process through planned and systematic activities. There are four important components in a quality management system: quality planning, quality control programme, quality assurance and quality improvement. The quality planning defines the quality criteria and provides the resources. The quality control programme provides the means to monitor and check the result of the process against the quality parameters. Quality control is the observation techniques and activities that are used to fulfil requirements for quality. Quality assurance is the planned and systematic activities in a quality system so that the quality requirement for a programme or system is ensured. Quality assurance is achieved through continuous evaluation of quality control activities at every step in the process and implementing the corrective measures. Quality improvement provides opportunity for improving the system based on experience and feedback. Unanticipated problems can be redressed through quality management system.

Good Pharmacovigilance Practices (GPvP) are set of measures required to facilitate the performance of pharmacovigilance system. A quality system in place would ensure good pharmacovigilance practices. GPvP guidelines describe how to establish a quality system in pharmacovigilance to ensure quality. GPvP is based on acquiring complete data from spontaneous adverse event reports (also called case reports). A good report should have at least the following elements:

- Description of adverse events;
- Details of suspected drug and concomitant drug therapy;
- Patient details;
- Details of diagnosis of events;
- Therapeutic measures and laboratory data at base line, during therapy and subsequent to therapy; and
- Details of de-challenge or re-challenge.

The regulatory authorities of US, UK etc., have issued GPvP guidance documents for adoption by pharmaceutical industries.

While it is beyond the scope of this chapter to discuss all aspects of quality system, three important issues are discussed: quality issues of data, audit programme of activities and assessing the programme.

I. *Quality of Data*:

In spite of introduction of active pharmacovigilance activities, the spontaneous reporting continues to be the main data source for pharmacovigilance activities. The whole process of data collection to retrieval and analysis must have rigorous procedure to ensure the best possible quality data. The management of data is also equally important.

There must be formal process and procedure [Standard Operating Procedure] in place to ensure the accuracy and completeness of the data. Data quality is based on/assessed by consistency in contents and nomenclature, level of details, data entry process, accuracy, relevance and completeness. .

II. *Pharmacovigilance Audit*:

Pharmacovigilance audit activities meant to verify, by examination and evaluation of objective evidence, the appropriateness and effectiveness of the implementation and operation of a pharmacovigilance system, including its quality system for pharmacovigilance activities.

In general, an audit is a systematic, disciplined, independent and documented process for obtaining evidence and evaluating the evidence objectively to determine the extent to which the audit criteria are fulfilled, contributing to the improvement of risk management, control and governance processes. Audit evidence consists of records, statements or other information, which are relevant to the audit criteria and verifiable. Audit criteria are, for each audit objective, the standards of performance and control against which the auditee and its activities will be assessed. In the context of pharmacovigilance, audit criteria should reflect the requirements for the pharmacovigilance system, including its quality system for pharmacovigilance activities, as found in the legislation and guidance.

A. The risk-based approach to pharmacovigilance audits

A risk-based approach is one that uses techniques to determine the areas of risk, where risk is defined as the probability of an event occurring that will have an impact on the achievement of objectives, taking account of the severity of its outcome and/or likelihood of non-detection by other methods. The risk-based approach to audits focuses on the areas of highest risk to the organisation's pharmacovigilance system, including its quality system for pharmacovigilance activities. In the context of pharmacovigilance, the risk to public health is of prime importance. Risk can be assessed at the following stages:

- Long term audit planning resulting in an audit strategy (long term approach), which should be endorsed by upper management;

- Short term audit planning resulting in an audit programme, setting audit objectives, and the extent and boundaries, often termed as scope, of the audits in that programme; and
- Operational level audit planning resulting in an audit plan for individual audit engagements, prioritising audit tasks based on risk and utilising risk-based sampling and testing approaches, and reporting of audit findings in line with their relative risk level and audit recommendations in line with the suggested grading system

Risk assessment should be documented appropriately for the long term, short term and operational planning of pharmacovigilance audit activity in the organisation

(a) ***Long term audit planning*****:** A high level statement of how the audit activities will be delivered over a period of time, longer than the annual programme, usually for a period of 2-5 years. The audit strategy includes a list of audits that could reasonably be performed. The audit strategy is used to outline the areas highlighted for audit, the audit topics as well as the methods and assumptions (including e.g., risk assessment) on which the audit programme is based.

The audit strategy should cover the governance, risk management and internal controls of all parts of the pharmacovigilance system including:

- All pharmacovigilance processes and tasks;
- The quality system for pharmacovigilance activities;
- Interactions and interfaces with other departments, as appropriate;
- Pharmacovigilance activities conducted by affiliated organisations or activities delegated to another organisation (e.g., regional reporting centres, MAH affiliates or third parties, such as contract organisations and other vendors).

This is a non-prioritised, non-exhaustive list of examples of risk factors that could be considered for the purposes of a risk assessment:

- Changes to legislation and guidance;
- Major re-organisation or other re-structuring of the pharmacovigilance system, mergers, acquisitions

(specifically for marketing authorisation holders, this may lead to a significant increase in the number of products for which the system is used);

- Change in key managerial function(s);
- Risk to availability of adequately trained and experienced pharmacovigilance staff, e.g. due to significant turn-over of staff, deficiencies in training processes, re-organisation, increase in volumes of work;
- Significant changes to the system since the time of a previous audit, e.g. introduction of a new database(s) for pharmacovigilance activities or of a significant upgrade to the existing database(s), changes to processes and activities in order to address new or amended regulatory requirements;
- First medicinal product on the market (for a marketing authorisation holder);
- Medicinal product(s) on the market with specific risk minimisation measures or other specific safety conditions such as requirements for additional monitoring;
- Criticality of the process, e.g., how critical is the area/process to proper functioning of the pharmaco-vigilance system. When deciding when to audit an affiliate or third party, the marketing authorisation holder should consider the nature and criticality of the pharmacovigilance activities that are being performed by an affiliate or third party on behalf of the marketing authorisation holder, in addition to considering the other factors included in this list;

Outcome of previous audits, e.g., has the area/process ever been audited (if not, then this may need to be prioritised depending on criticality); if the area/process has previously been audited, the audit findings* are a factor to consider when deciding when to re-audit the area/process, including the implementation of agreed actions;

- Identified procedural gaps relating to specific areas/ processes;
- Other organisational changes that could negatively impact on the area/process, e.g., if a change occurs to a

support function (such as information technology support) this could negatively impact upon pharmacovigilance activities.

(b) ***Short term audit planning***: An audit programme is a set of one or more audits planned for a specific timeframe, normally for a year. It should be prepared in line with the long term audit strategy. The audit programme should be approved by upper management with overall responsibility for operational and governance structure.

The risk-based audit programme should be based on an appropriate risk assessment and should focus on:

- The quality system for pharmacovigilance activities;
- Critical pharmacovigilance processes;
- Key control systems relied on for pharmacovigilance activities;
- Areas identified as high risk, after controls have been put in place or mitigating action taken.

The risk-based audit programme should also take into account historical areas with insufficient past audit coverage, and high risk areas identified by and/or specific requests from management and/or persons responsible for pharmacovigilance activities.

The audit programme documentation should include a brief description of the plan for each audit to be delivered, including an outline of scope and objectives.

The rationale for the timing, periodicity and scope of the individual audits which form part of the audit programme should be based on the documented risk assessment. However, risk-based pharmacovigilance audit(s) should be performed at regular intervals, which are in line with legislative requirements.

Changes to the audit programme may happen and will require proper documentation.

(c) ***Operational level audit planning and reporting***

(i) ***Planning and fieldwork***: The organisation should ensure that written procedures are in place regarding the planning and conduct of individual audits that will be delivered. Timeframes for all the steps required for the performance of an individual audit should be settled in the relevant audit related procedures, and the organisation should ensure that audits are conducted in accordance with the written procedures, in line with applicable regulation of that country.

Individual pharmacovigilance audits should be undertaken in line with the approved risk-based audit programme. When planning individual audits, the auditor identifies and assesses the risks relevant to the area under review and employs the most appropriate risk-based sampling and testing methods, documenting the audit approach in an audit plan.

(ii) ***Audit reporting*:** The findings of the auditors should be documented in an audit report and should be communicated to management in a timely manner. The audit process should include mechanisms for communicating the audit findings to the auditee and receiving feedback, and reporting the audit findings to management and relevant parties, including those responsible for pharmacovigilance systems, in accordance with legal requirements and guidance on pharmacovigilance audits. Audit findings should be reported in line with their relative risk level and should be graded in order to indicate their relative criticality to risks impacting the pharmacovigilance system, processes and parts of processes. The grading system should be defined in the description of the quality system for pharmacovigilance, and should take into consideration the thresholds noted below which would be used in further reporting:

- ***Critical*** is a fundamental weakness in one or more pharmacovigilance processes or practices that adversely affects the whole pharmacovigilance system and/or the rights, safety or well-being of patients, or that poses a potential risk to public health and/or represents a serious violation of applicable regulatory requirements.
- ***Major*** is a significant weakness in one or more pharmacovigilance processes or practices, or a

fundamental weakness in part of one or more pharmacovigilance processes or practices that is detrimental to the whole process and/or could potentially adversely affect the rights, safety or well-being of patients and/or could potentially pose a risk to public health and/or represents a violation of applicable regulatory requirements which is however not considered serious.

- ***Minor*** is a weakness in the part of one or more pharmacovigilance processes or practices that is not expected to adversely affect the whole pharmacovigilance system or process and/or the rights, safety or well-being of patients.

  Issues that need to be urgently addressed should be communicated in an expedited manner to the auditee's management and the upper management.

(iii) *Actions based on audit outcomes and follow-up of audits:*

Actions: immediate action, prompt action, action within a reasonable timeframe, issues that need to be urgently addressed, or communicated in an expedited manner, are intended to convey timelines that are appropriate, relevant, and in line with the relative risk to the pharmacovigilance system.

Corrective and preventive actions to address critical and major issues should be prioritised. The precise timeframe for action(s) related to a given critical finding, for example, may differ depending on nature of findings and the planned action(s).

The management of the organisation is responsible for ensuring that the organisation has a mechanism in place to adequately address the issues arising from pharmacovigilance audits. Actions should include root cause analysis and impact analysis of identified audit findings and preparation of a corrective and preventive action plan, where appropriate.

Upper management and those charged with governance, should ensure that effective action is implemented to address the audit findings. The implementation of agreed actions should be monitored in a systematic way, and the progress of implementation should be communicated on a periodic basis proportionate to the planned actions to upper management.

Evidence of completion of actions should be recorded in order to document that issues raised during the audit have been addressed.

Capacity for follow-up audits should be foreseen in the audit programme. They should be carried out as deemed necessary, in order to verify the completion of agreed actions.

(iv) ***Quality system and record management practices:***

The organisation should assign the specific responsibilities for the pharmacovigilance audit activities. Pharmacovigilance audit activities should be independent. The organisation's management should ensure this independence and objectivity in a structured manner and document this.

Auditors should be free from interference in determining the scope of auditing, performing pharmacovigilance audits and communicating audit results. The main reporting line should be to the upper management with overall responsibility for operational and governance structure that allows the auditor(s) to fulfil their responsibilities and to provide independent, objective audit opinion. Auditors can consult with technical experts, personnel involved in pharmacovigilance processes, and with the person responsible for pharmacovigilance; however auditors should maintain an unbiased attitude that allows them to perform audit work in such a manner that they have an honest belief in their work product and that no significant quality compromises are made. Objectivity requires auditors not to subordinate their judgement on audit matters to that of others.

(v) ***Qualifications, skills and experience of auditors and continuing professional development:*** Auditors should demonstrate and maintain proficiency in terms of the knowledge, skills and abilities required to effectively conduct and/or participate in pharmacovigilance audit activities. The proficiency of audit team members will have been gained through a combination of education, work experience and training and, as a team, should cover knowledge, skills and abilities in:

- Audit principles, procedures and techniques;
- Applicable laws, regulations and other requirements relevant to pharmacovigilance;
- Pharmacovigilance activities, processes and system(s);
- Management system(s);
- Organisational system(s).

(vi) ***Evaluation of the quality of audit activities:*** Evaluation of audit work can be undertaken by means of ongoing and periodic assessment of all audit activities, auditee feedback and self-assessment of audit activities (e.g., quality assurance of audit activities, compliance to code of conduct, audit programme, and audit procedures).

(vii) ***Audits undertaken by outsourced audit service providers:*** Ultimate responsibility for the operation and effectiveness of the pharmacovigilance system resides within the organisation. Where the organisation decides to use an outsourced audit service provider to implement the pharmacovigilance audit requirements on the basis of applicable regulation and perform pharmacovigilance audits:

- The requirements and preparation of the audit risk assessment, the audit strategy and audit programme and individual engagements should be specified to the outsourced service providers, by the organisation, in writing;
- The scope, objectives and procedural requirements for the audit should be specified to the outsourced service provider, by the organisation, in writing;
- The organisation should obtain and document assurance of the independence and objectivity of outsourced service providers;
- The outsourced audit service provider should also follow the relevant regulatory requirement.

III. *Assessment of Pharmacovigilance System*:

It is always necessary to assess a system in order to ensure that the system functions in the expected way. The evaluation of data collection practice, analysis of data and interpretation of data at different level of the system would help develop recommendations and identify priority interventions to improve the critical aspects of pharmacovigilance system. The outcome of a pharmacovigilance system should be reduction in medicine related problems. Management Sciences for Health, USA, has developed 43 indicators that address the following five components:

(a) Policy, law and regulation;

(b) Systems, structures, and stake holders coordination;

(c) Signal generation and data management;

(d) Risk assessment and evaluation; and

(e) Risk management and communication.

There are 26 core indicators and 17 supplementary indicators. Core indictors are important and essential. The core indicators with their importance are given in the table given below. The readers are encouraged to refer the original publication to learn about the supplementary indictors.

S. No.	Indicator	What for Used	Frequency of Assessment
Policy, Law and Regulation			
1	Existence of a policy document that contains essential statements on pharmacovigilance (stand alone or as a part of some other policy document)	Structural	Every five years
2	Existence of specific legal provisions for pharmacovigilance in the national medicines legislation or similar legislation	Structural	Every five years
Systems, Structures, and Stakeholder Coordination			
3	Existence of a pharmacovigilance center or unit	Structural	Every five years
4	Pharmacovigilance center or unit has a clear mandate, structure, roles, and responsibilities	Structural	Every five years

Contd...

S. No.	Indicator	What for Used	Frequency of Assessment
5	Existence of a medicine information or pharmacovigilance service that provides ADR and drug safety–related question-and-answer services	Structural	Annually
6	A designated staff responsible for pharmacovigilance or medicine safety activities	Structural	Annually
7	Dedicated budget available for pharmacovigilance-related activities	Structural	Annually
8	Existence of a national medicine safety advisory committee or a subcommittee with similar functions that has met at least once in the last year	Structural	Annually
9	Existence of national pharma-covigilance guidelines updated within the last five years	Structural	Every five years
10	Existence of protocols or SOPs for improving patient safety relating to medicine use	Structural	Annually
11	Existence of a minimum core list of communication technologies to improve access to safety reporting and provision of medicine information	Structural	Annually
12	Existence of an ADR or medicine safety bulletin (or any other health-related newsletter that routinely features ADR or medicine safety issues) published in the last six months	Structural	Annually
13	Platform or strategy exists for the coordination of pharmacovigilance activities at the national level	Structural	Annually
Signal Generation and Data Management			
14	Existence of a system for coordination and collation of pharmacovigilance data from all sources in the country (e.g., health programs, immunization program, active surveillance studies)	Process	Annually
15	Existence of a database for tracking pharmacovigilance activities	Process	Annually

Contd...

S. No.	Indicator	What for Used	Frequency of Assessment
16	Existence of a form for reporting suspected ADRs	Process	Annually
17	Existence of a form for reporting suspected product quality issues (as a subset in the ADR form or as a separate form)	Process	Annually
18	Existence of a form for reporting suspected medication errors (as a subset in the ADR form or as a separate form)	Process	Annually
19	Existence of a form for reporting suspected treatment failure (as a subset in the ADR form or as a separate form)	Process	Annually
	Risk Assessment and Evaluation		
20	Number of ADR reports received in the last year	Process	Annually
21	Number of active surveillance activities currently ongoing or carried out in the last five years	Process	Every five years
22	Percentage of patients in public health programs for whom drug-related adverse events were reported in the last year (disaggregated by type of adverse event, drug, severity, outcomes, and demographics)	Process	Annually
23	Percentage of patients under going treatment within a public health program whose treatment was modified because of treatment failure or ADRs in the last year (disaggregated by treatment failure and ADRs)	Process	Annually
	Risk Management and Communication		
24	Average time lag between identification of safety signal of a serious ADR or significant medicine safety issue and communication to health care workers and the public	Outcome	Annually

Contd...

S. No.	Indicator	What for Used	Frequency of Assessment
25	Percentage of the sampled Drug and Therapeutics Committees that have carried out pharmacovigilance activities or addressed medicine safety issues in the last year	Outcome	Annually
26	Percentage of medicines sampled in the last year that passed product quality tests	Outcome	Annually

The national medicine regulatory authority, public health programmes, health facilities and researchers concerned with pharmacovigilance can utilize these tools to assess the various segments of pharmacovigilance systems: structure, process and outcome.

Key Messages

- Quality control is the observation techniques and activities that are used to fulfil requirements for quality. Quality assurance is the planned and systematic activities implemented in a quality system to ensure quality requirements in a product or process. In general, quality assurance defines the standards to be followed in order to meet the requirements while quality control ensures that these standards are followed at every step.
- Good Pharmacovigilance Practices (GPvP) are set of measures required to facilitate the performance of pharmacovigilance system. A quality system in place would ensure good pharmacovigilance practices.
- Three important components of quality system: quality of data, auditing and periodic assessment of the programme.
- Quality of data focuses on good case report.
- Auditing verifies, through objective evidence, the appropriateness and effectiveness of the implementation and operation of a pharmacovigilance system including its quality system for pharmacovigilance activities.
- The evaluation of data collection practice, analysis of data and interpretation of data at different level of the system would help develop recommendations and identify priority interventions to improve the critical aspects of pharmacovigilance system. The indictor based assessment facilitates evaluation.

Bibliography

1. Guideline on good pharmacovigilance practices, EMA/541760/2011 Dated 22 June 2012, European Medicine Agency.
2. Marie Lindquist, Data Quality Management in Pharmacovigilance, Drug Safety, 27(12), 2004.
3. Indicator Based Pharmacovigilance Assessment Tool: Manual for Conducting Assessments in Developing Countries, Management Sciences for Health, December 2009.

[Contributed by Mr. Shaikh Ruhu Al Amin]

Chapter 8

Periodic Safety Update Reports

"The death of one man is a tragedy. The death of millions is a statistic".

Joe Stalin, comment to Churchill at Potsdam, 1945

After reading this chapter, you should be able to understand and appreciate:
• Concept of Periodic Safety Update Reports [PSURs]; • Components of PSURs; • How to develop PSURs and • PSURs provisions of India, UK and USA.

Many medicinal/pharmaceutical products have been withdrawn from various markets over the years because of actual or perceived safety issues. It is estimated that one-third of them were withdrawn within two years of launch and half within five years. Withdrawal of products after marketing approval substantiate the need of submission of post marketing surveillance report of all approved drugs to the medicine regulatory authorities. The clinical trials in limited number of patients and in controlled condition cannot detect all possible adverse drug reactions. Many new adverse drug reactions are detected when drugs are in use in real world: large population, different co-morbid conditions and along with other drugs. Hence, the regulatory authorities throughout the world require that the marketing authorization holder (pharmaceutical company marketing the medicinal product) needs submitting the safety report periodically after marketing approval. This requirement is also known as post marketing surveillance. The submission of safety update reports periodically is called Periodic Safety Update Reports (PSURs).

The PSURs are defined as systematic review of global safety data which became available to the marketing authorization holder of a marketed medicinal product at predefined time interval. The purpose of the PSURs is to provide a comprehensive and critical analysis of risk-benefit balance of a medicinal product taking into account of new or emerging information in the cumulative risk-benefit analysis. The frequency of submission of the PSURs is usually mentioned in the marketing authorization. In general routine PSURs are not required for products of low risks like well established medicinal products and generics.

There are two main stake holders on PSUR: the companies who develop the PSUR and submit to the Regulatory Authority; and the Regulatory Authority who reviews the report and take regulatory decision. PSURs provide opportunities for the marketing authorization holder to review the safety profile of their products and ensure that summary of product characteristics and patient information leaflets are up to date. On the other hand, the quality of PSURs is a good indicator of overall state of Pharmacovigilance system of marketing authorization holders. For drug regulatory authorities, PSURs are valuable Pharmacovigilance data to initiate regulatory decisions including banning a product.

In general PSUR begins with approval of medicinal product and continues for the entire marketing life of the product.

Periodicity: PSURs are not cumulative documents. They cover a predefined period which is specified by the regulatory authority. The frequency or periodicity varies from country to country. In European Union, the requirements are: six monthly PSURs for first two years, annual reports for next two years, and then five years report thereafter. In Japan, PSUR requirement for new chemical entity is every six months for two years and annually for next four years. For new formulation, PSUR is required for every six months for two years and then annually for next two years.

Content and format: Worldwide there are attempts to simplify the procedure as well as to make uniform format for submission of PSURs. The following is the basic structure of a PSUR:

- Executive Summary
- Introduction or scope of the report

- Worldwide marketing authorization status
- Action taken for safety reason and changes to core safety information
- Patient exposure data
- Individual case histories
- Information from formal studies
- Overall safety evaluation [important and newly identified or ongoing safety issues are documented and proposals to address them]
- Important information received after the data lock period (cut off date) or last report
- Core safety information

Each product is usually assigned an international birth date (IBD), the day of first approval anywhere in the world. This is the basis of cut off dates for submission of reports.

The readers are encouraged to see the prototype reports in Current Challenges in Pharmacovigilance: Pragmatic Approaches, Report of CIOMS working V, Geneva 2001 [http://www.cioms.ch/index.php/component/booklibrary/?task=view&Itemid=&id=47&catid=58].

PSUR in India: Indian regulation [Schedule Y of Drugs and Cosmetics Rules under Drugs and Cosmetics Act] requires that PSURs of new drugs are required to be submitted to the office of DCG (I) every six months for the first two years and thereafter annually for next two years. The PSURs due for the period must be submitted within 30 calendar days of the last day of the report. The manufacturers or importers are responsible for complying with this legal obligation.

The report should be India specific and must be structured to contain the followings:

1. A title page stating: Periodic Safety Update Report for the product, applicants name, period covered by the report, date of approval of the new drug, approved indication, date of marketing of new drug and date of reporting;
2. Introduction;
3. Current worldwide market authorization status;
4. Update of action taken for safety reasons;
5. Changes to reference safety information;

6. Estimated patient exposure;
7. Presentation of individual case histories;
8. Studies;
9. Other Information;
10. Overall safety evaluation;
11. Conclusion; and
12. Appendix providing material relating to indications, dosing, pharmacology and other related information.

Though PSURs are mandatory, the pharmaceutical companies do not comply with this requirement. This is evident from the report of Parliamentary Standing Committee on Health and Family Welfare [59th Report on Functioning of CDSCO, 2012]. The Committee observed that there was not only non-compliance on submission of reports but also the reports were neither India specific nor in appropriate format. The Committee strongly recommended the Ministry to warn the manufacturers of new drugs to comply with mandatory provision of PSURs or face suspension of marketing approval.

The Government of India now proposes to direct the pharmaceutical companies to have pharmacovigilance system to periodically submit safety update reports to the CDSCO, the central regulatory agency on Drugs and Medical Devices. The National Coordinating Centre of Pharmacovigilance Programme of India, Indian Pharmacopoeia Commission, too plans to set up dedicated cell to start work on reviewing the PSURs as Government plans to link PSURs to Pharmacovigilance Programme.

***PSUR in USA*:** US FDA issued new guideline titled "Providing post-market periodic safety reports in the ICH E2C (R2) format [Periodic Benefit – Risk Evaluation Report (PBRER)]". PBRER replaced the earlier format of submitting PSURs as Periodic Adverse Drug Experience Report (PADER) or Periodic Adverse Experience Report (PAER) or PSUR. However, the pharmaceutical companies (Marketing Authorization Holder) may seek waiver of PBRER and submit the PSUR in earlier format. PBRER is in consistent with latest ICH requirements. The reports are to be submitted quarterly for the first three years following US approval and annually thereafter.

***PSUR in United Kingdom*:** The PSURs are replaced by periodic benefit risk evaluation report (PBRER). The PBRER is a periodic assessment of the risk-benefit balance of a medicinal product. The marketing authorization holder needs to submit the report irrespective of the product is in the market or not. The PBRER provides an analysis of safety, efficacy and effectiveness of the product in the entire life cycle. The report submission periodicity: every six months until the product is placed in the market, every six months for the first two years of introducing the product into the market and annually for the next two years.

Routine PBRERs are not required if the medicinal products fall under the EU's directives. These are: Generics, Products with well established use, Homeopathic medicines and Traditional herbal medicines. PBRERs are jointly assessed by the Medicines and Healthcare Products Regulatory Agency (MHRA) and other European national competent authorities assigned by Pharmacovigilance Risk Assessment Committee (PRAC) or a member country appointed by the Coordination Group for Mutual recognition and Decentralised Procedures. The PRAC issues recommendations for PBRERs for: a centrally authorized product, any mix of centrally authorized products and those under National and EU procedures, and nationally authorised products reflected in the European Union Reference Data (EURD) list. MHRA assesses products for active substances authorized in UK only on an individual basis.

Key Messages

- Submissions of PSURs are post marketing obligations of marketing authorization holders.
- PSURs are systematic review of global safety data which became available to the marketing authorization holders of a marketed medicinal product at pre-defined time interval.
- PSURs are helpful for the marketing authorization holder to ensure the updated product characteristics and patient information leaflets.
- PSURs are valuable Pharmacovigilance data for regulatory authorities to initiate decisions including restricting use or banning a product.
- PSUR begins with approval of the medicinal product and continues for the entire life cycle. The PSURS are to be developed and submitted at predefined time interval as desired by the corresponding regulatory authority.
- Content and format for PSUR are not uniform worldwide. However, ICH guideline E2C (R2) is widely accepted.
- Schedule Y of Drugs and Cosmetics Rule of Drugs and Cosmetics Act (India) specifies the periodicity and format for submission of PSURs.
- Periodic Benefit Risk Evaluation Report has replaced the traditional PSURs in USA and UK and is in consistent of ICH guidelines.

Bibliography

1. 59th Report on the Functioning of the Central Drugs Control Organization, Parliamentary Standing Committee on Health and Family Welfare, 2012.
2. Good Pharmacovigilance Practice Guide, Compiled by the Medicines and healthcare Products Regulatory Agency, Pharmaceutical Press, 2010.
3. Current Challenges in Pharmacovigilance: Pragmatic Approaches, Reports of CIOMS Working Group V, CIOMS, 2001.
4. Medicines, medical devices and blood regulation and safety guidance, Periodic benefit risk evaluation reports for medicinal products, 18 December 2014, accessed at https://www.gov.uk/periodic-benefit-risk-evaluation-reports-for-medicinal-products on 8 May 2015.
5. Guidance for Industry, Providing Postmarket periodic Safety Reports in the ICH E2C (R2) Format, Periodic Benefit-Risk Evaluation Report, Draft Guidance, US Department of Health and Human Services, Food and Drug Administration, Centre for Drug evaluation and Research, Centre for Biologics Evaluation and Research, April 2013, accessed at http://www.fda.gov/downloads/drugs/guidancecomplianceregulatoryinformation/guidances/ucm346564.pdf on 08 May 2015.
6. Guru Prasad Mohanta, Textbook on Clinical Research: A Guide for Aspiring Professionals and Professionals, PharmaMed Press, 2011.

Chapter 9

Pharmacogenetics in Pharmacovigilance

"The only true wisdom is knowing you know nothing".

Socrates

After reading this chapter, you should be able to understand and appreciate:
• Why different persons respond to medicines differently. • Influence of genetic variations in medicine action especially causing ADRs. • Generic markers as risk indicators. • Classical examples showing genetic basis of ADRs. • Importance of Pharmacogenetics ensuring safe and more effective medicines.

The inter–individual variability in response to medication is well known. The genetic factors that affect the kinetics and dynamics of medicines play a greater role in determining the individual's risk of non-response or toxicity. Genes affect the way in which the body processes and responds to drugs. Genetic differences explain some of the inter-individual variability in patients' response to some medicines. The variation in gene coding for drug metabolizing enzymes, drug transporters, drug receptors and targets account for a significant portion of the observed heterogeneity in drug response across population. The study of genetically determined variations in drug response is called Pharmacogenetics. In addition to the genetic polymorphism, there are many factors which are responsible for variation in drug response: age of the patient, size – weight and height or body mass index, pregnancy, co-morbidity and renal or liver damage.

Adverse Effects of Codeine

CYP2D6 genotype influences the response to codeine. Poor metabolisers do not convert codeine efficiently to morphine and they get little analgesic effect from codeine. On the other hand, ultra-rapid metabolisers may experience morphine toxicity. High level of morphine can result in breathing difficulty, which may be fatal. 5-10% of Caucasians (human race of Europe, Western Asia, parts of India and North Africa) are poor metabolisers. 29% of North African and Ethiopian populations are ultra-rapid metabolizers and about 6 percent of African American, Caucasian and Greek populations too have similar issues.

Codeine related deaths in children following tonsillectomy have been linked to ultra-rapid metabolism. Children were given codeine for pain relief after surgery that resulted in death of few children [2012]. The adverse drug reporting system of USFDA identified 10 deaths and three over dosage associated with codeine during 1969 to 2012. The USFDA has issued a black box warning for codeine use in children after tonsillectomy.

While it is difficult to know the metabolising status of the individual without genetic testing, it is preferable not to use codeine in children following tonsil removal and to use alternatives for pain management. CYP2D6 genotyping is not routine before prescribing codeine.

The genetically based variations in drug response are primarily caused by mutations of DNA, which result in structural changes of proteins involved in different pharmacokinetic phases of absorption, distribution, metabolism and elimination as well as in drug receptor interactions. Much of the individual's pharmacogenetic response is attributed to the difference in metabolism called genetic polymorphism. The genetic polymorphism is the inter-individual differences in DNA sequences at a specific chromosomal location that exist at a frequency of more than 1% at general population. The two alleles (alternate form of genes) at a given gene locus comprise the genotype. The influence of genotype on phenotype is measurable. The genotype is the genetic code in the cell and the phenotype is the expression and observable traits. Though pharmacognetics have wide application in medical sciences, this chapter restricts the discussion related to Adverse Drug Reactions.

The effect of age on the impact of genetic polymorphism should be considered. The enzyme and transport proteins involved in the pharmacokinetic of a drug may be different in young paediatric patients than in adults as a consequence of different regulation of gene expression. Such differences are mainly expected in new born infants, infants and toddler. There is expression of CYP3A7 in new born and post natal increase in CYP2C9, 2C19 and 3A4 expression in the first year after birth. When a significant impact of a genetic polymorphism on the pharmacokinetics of a drug and/or risk of adverse drug reaction has been established in adults, the potential consequences in the paediatric population should also be considered.

Genetic susceptibility to Adverse Drug Reactions has been established for a number of drugs. Some clinically significant issues are narrated below. Of the CYP enzymes involved in drug metabolism, CYP2C9, CYP2C19 and CYP2D6 are polymorphically expressed clinically important enzymes. The CYP2D6 poor metaboliser phenotype is found in 5-10% of Caucasians and North Americans of African descent and about 1-2% of Asian subjects. The molecular basis for lack of CYP2D6 is explainable. With the present genotyping technologies, CYP2D6 poor metabolisers can be easily identified. The poor metaboliser phenotype for CYP2D6 is reported to cause insufficient metabolism in many therapeutic classes. CYP2C19 (or, mephenytoin hydroxylase) deficiency is found in 3-5% of the Caucasian population and in about 20% of the Asian population.

Warfarin and Genetic Variation

Warfarin reduces blood's ability to clot and prevents blood clots in vein, arteries and heart. It acts by blocking the liver's production of certain clotting factors and has been extensively used in deep venous thrombosis, pulmonary embolus, and in atrial fibrillation. The dose of warfarin needs to be closely monitored and adjusted to achieve appropriate balance between the anti-clotting benefits and serious risk of life threatening bleeding. The two genes are found to influence the effect of warfarin. The gene CYP2C9 is used by the liver cells to make an enzyme that breaks down warfarin. Because of variation in gene type some people metabolise warfarin more slowly than others. Patients with this gene variant (slow metabolisers) require less warfarin to achieve the same anti-clotting effect. With the same normal dose, these patients experience toxicity. The variant of second gene, VKORC1 (Vitamin K epoxide reductase), cause patients to have increased sensitivity to warfarin and requires lower dosing. Vitamin K obtained from diet or vitamin supplements interferes with warfarin. Vitamin K helps the blood clot. Genetic variation in the VKORC1 influences warfarin dosing by three fold than CYP2C9. Realizing the influence of genetic variation in safe warfarin therapy, USFDA (2007) encouraged genetic tests for appropriate dosing. However, recent studies reported in New England Journal of Medicine

(2013) provide strong evidence that genetic testing of warfarin responsiveness does not provide any meaningful benefit to patients being started with warfarin.

Hypersensitivity Syndrome of Abacavir

Abacavir is a nucleoside analogue used in the treatment of AIDS. About 5-9% of the patients develop hypersensitive reactions of which 94% develop the reactions in first 6 weeks of treatment. The hypersensitive reactions are: skin rash, gastrointestinal and respiratory (dyspnea, cough, and pharyngitis) manifestations and re-challenge shock. Failure to recognise these reactions and continued treatment is associated with fatalities. The treatment for these reactions is to stop using abacavir. Re-treatment with abacavir can cause serious allergic reactions including anaphylactic shock.

The study has shown that several genetic markers are associated with abacavir hypersensitivity. But HLA-B*5701 alone serves as an excellent predictive abacavir hypersensitivity syndrome. There is lower risk of hypersensitivity in blacks but it is preferable to screen both black and white population. It is recommended that screening of HLA-B*5701 before starting any abacavir containing regimen on any patient. A positive test indicates that the person is susceptible and the drug should not be given. Though HLA-B*5701 is an excellent tool for detecting abacavir hypersensitivity, the negative test result does not absolutely rule out hypersensitivity. The genetic test is conducted in blood or saliva sample.

Aspirin Adverse Effects

Aspirin has been widely used at low dose to prevent cardiovascular events due to its anti-platelet activity. A new research claims that the common genetic variation in the gene for catechol-O-methyltransferase (COMT) may alter the action of aspirin and harm the persons. COMT is a key enzyme in the metabolism of catecholamines (epinephrine, norepinephrine, and dopamine). These hormones have good influence in hypertension. The study reported that individuals who are homozygous for the enzyme's high-activity valine form, the "val/vals," have been shown to have lower levels of catecholamines compared to individuals who are homozygous for the enzyme's low-activity methionine form, the "met/mets". It is found that the 23% of the women who were 'val/vals' were naturally protected against incident cardiovascular disease.

However, when the women with the val/val polymorphism were allocated aspirin, this natural protection was eliminated. The study showed that val/val women who were randomly assigned aspirin had more cardiovascular events than the val/vals who were assigned placebo; while women, who were met/met, had fewer cardiovascular events when assigned aspirin compared to placebo.

As COMT genetic variant is very common, it may be necessary to individualize the therapy based on genetic profile.

Clopidogrel Adverse Effects

Clopidogrel is used to prevent serious or life threatening problems with the heart and blood vessels in people who had stroke, heart attack, or severe chest pain. It works by preventing platelets from collecting and forming clots that may cause stroke or heart attack. This is a prodrug which is metabolised mainly by CYP2C19 to produce active metabolite that inhibits platelet aggregation. In patients who are CYP2C19 poor metaboliser, less of active metabolite is formed which may result in serious clinical implications: stent thrombosis, myocardial infarction or even death. Based on study reports, the product information of Clopidogrel was updated in European Union to include information related to an increased risk of cardiovascular events with reduced CYP2C19 function due to genetic variant in the gene coding for the CYP2C19 protein. Similar safety concern is also an issue when Clopidogrel is used with CYP2C19 inhibitors like proton pump inhibitors.

Some Clinically significant Adverse Drug Response associated with pharmacogenetics.

Drug	Adverse Response	Responsible Polymorphic Gene
Warfarin (for preventing blood cloting)	Haemorrhage in poor metabolisers	CYP2C9
Irinotecan (for colon or rectal cancer)	Neutropenia	UGT1A1*28
Albuterol (for asthma and COPD)	Asthma control result is based on argino geno type or glycine geno type	β2 Adrenergic receptor
Pravastatin (for cholesterol lowering)	Reduced cholesterol lowering response	CETP

Contd...

Drug	Adverse Response	Responsible Polymorphic Gene
Zileuton (Leukotriene synthesis inhibitor used in asthma)	Variation in response	5-Lipoxygenase
Abacavir (for HIV)	Hypersensitivity	HLA-B*5701
Primaquine (for Malaria)	Haemolytic anaemia (in deficient enzyme patients)	G6PD
Azathioprine (for prevention of treatment rejection and severe rheumatoid arthritis)	Myelosuppression (TPM deficient patients accumulate excessive thioguanine nucleotide)	Thiopurine S-methyltransferase (TPM)
6-mercaptopurine (for acute lymphocytic leukaemia)	Neutropenia and other toxicity	TPMT*2, *3A, *3B, *3C
Gefitnib (for lung cancer)	Diarrhoea	ABCG2Q141K
Isoniazid (for TB)	Hepatotoxic	CYP2E1*1 and NAT2
Tranilast (anti-allergic)	Hyper-bilirubinemia	UGT1A1*28
Allopurinol (for Gout)	Severe Cutaneous	HLA-B*5801
Carbamazepine (for seizure)	Steven Johnson Syndrome (highest risk in persons of Asian Ancestry)	HLA-B*1502

Valuable information can be generated from well documented case reports including information on the relationship between biomarkers (geno type or pheno type) and the clinical features of adverse drug reactions. Spontaneous ADR reports related to possible genetic polymorphism could be the important data source for signal generation or risk evaluation. Well documented case reports may lead to product information change and/or trigger pharmacogenetic research. Description of genomic biomarker information in the product information is essential and the testing the patients may be essential. Medicine induced harm is a public health issue. The pharmacogenomics promise a clearer path to predicting in whom the harm is most likely to occur. Once predicted, it would ensure right medicine to right person thus promoting safety and efficacy. However, the evaluation of economic burden of the ADRs and the cost effectiveness of the pharmacogenetic tests is crucial.

Key Messages

- The variation in gene coding for drug metabolizing enzymes, drug transporters, drug receptors and targets contribute significantly for heterogeneity in drug response across population.
- The genetically based variations in drug response are primarily caused by mutation of DNA which affects pharmacokinetics and drug-receptor interactions. Much of the individual pharmacogenetic response is attributed due to difference in metabolism (genetic polymorphism).
- Genetic susceptibility to adverse drug reactions is established for a number of drugs.
- Spontaneous ADR reports related to genetic polymorphism is an important data source for signal generation or risk evaluation. Pharmacogenetic tests helps in identifying patients in whom the harm is most likely to occur.

Bibliography

1. Guideline on key aspects for use of pharmacogenomic methodologies in the Pharmacovigilance evaluation of medicinal products, Draft, European Medicine Agency, 2014.
2. Roger Walker and Cate Whittlesea, Clinical Pharmacy and Therapeutics, Fifth Edition, Churchil Livingstone, Elsevier, 2012.
3. Ronald D. Mann and Elizabeth B. Andrews (Editors), Pharmacovigilance, Second Edition, John Wiley and Sons, Ltd., 2007.

Chapter 10

Ethical Consideration in Pharmacovigilance

"One must educate the public that seldom does a patient receive the best treatment"

The Flexner Report

After reading this chapter, you should be able to understand and appreciate:
• Whether there is need of observing / complying with ethical requirements for biomedical research. • Main ethical issues.

Introduction

The medicines are essential for preventing and treating diseases or illnesses. They have harmful effects too. Until the medicines have been in use in diverse population over a long period of time, there are substantial uncertainties on benefit and risks of these medicines. The Pharmacovigilance activities are concerned with detection and documentation of these risks in an attempt to promote safe use of medicines. Regulatory authorities and pharmaceutical companies continue monitoring the drugs while they are in market. The patient and reporter identifiability are important requirements in Pharmacovigilance. They assure the existence of a real person that can be verified or validated in some way. Activities involving human subjects (patients) require ethical consideration.

Main bioethical principles: Ethical principles of biomedical research in human beings are mainly comprised of:

- Non- Maleficence (Do no harm);
- Beneficence (Fruitful result, Do good);
- Autonomy (Respect for persons); and
- Justice (Distributive justice, equitable distribution of risks and benefits).

The potential benefits to the participants, anticipated risks and the compensation thereof, unexpected consequences and the procedures proposed to tackle are covered under first two principles (Non-Maleficence and Beneficence). Informed consent, and privacy and confidentiality of the data are covered under the third point (Autonomy). The principles of justice require that the fruit of research is equitably shared amongst the beneficiaries and research participants. All clinical or biomedical research needs to comply with these requirements. They are the part of Good Clinical Practice guidelines.

Randomized control trials in post marketing phase: Safety monitoring of approved medicines may be broadly divided into two types: Post-Marketing Surveillance (Phase-IV of Clinical Trials, a responsibility of the pharmaceutical company) and routine documentation of adverse drug reaction (Pharmacovigilance programme of Drug Regulatory Authority). Post Marketing Research questions focus on drug's risk and such study designs provide safety evidence of sufficient quality for decision making. When post-marketing randomized control trials are conducted by the pharmaceutical companies, it is essential to protect patients' or participants' rights and interest. Post-Marketing Randomized Control Trials (RCT) are justified in the following conditions:

- A regulatory decision cannot be taken on the basis of available evidence or evidence that could be obtained through observational studies;
- RCTs can be properly designed and implemented to generate evidence for a responsible regulatory decision;
- The regulatory authority will use the trial results in making a regulatory decision in a timely manner; and
- RCT has provision to protect the rights and interest of participants.

Informed consent and confidentiality in PV: The Pharmacovigilance activities are neither clinical trials nor research activities (studies). They are just observational data collection activities without any intervention in the treatment. These activities are recognised as public health activities. As the PV activities are initiated by the Governments (Regulatory Authorities), the informed consent is not required for collection of data for safety monitoring. However, it is essential to maintain the security, privacy and confidentiality of personal data. Personal identifier is an important requirement of PV to avoid duplication and follow up, if required. As patient identifier is recorded, strict conditions are necessary on maintaining data security. Personal identifiable data of both patients and reporter should not be shared with any other parties including pharmaceutical companies or research groups. The published data including reports should not contain any information that could identify the patients.

The persons responsible for PV activities need to be trained in the strict maintenance of security and confidentiality.

Re-challenge: Perhaps the most powerful pieces of evidence to ascertain causality between adverse drug reaction and the suspected drug is the subsequent re-administration of the medicine. This is called re-challenge. It is a matter of debate whether it is appropriate to perform a re-challenge! A decision to re-administer the suspected drug causing adverse drug reaction is dependent on factors like whether the reaction is reversible, whether it is idiosyncratic etc. Careful judgement of the treating clinician is important. Patient informed consent is essential especially if the adverse reaction is serious or medically important. Re-challenge for scientific interest alone is not ethical. Intentional re-challenge should be carried out only when there is likely to be clinical benefit to the patient. This should be done when the treating physician is of the view that the anticipated result is directly relevant to the patient's treatment and well being.

Key Messages

- "Do no harm, Do good, Respect for persons and equitable distribution of risks and benefits" are the fundamental principles of bioethics.
- PV activities involve with minimal risks (almost nil) and hence ethical consideration is less.
- PV programme initiated by regulatory authority is accepted as public health practice not as research. Hence, does not require the necessity of informed consent.
- PMS (observational Studies) conducted by pharmaceutical companies – no clear guidance on the need of informed consent.

Contd...

- RCTs conducted as Phase – IV of Clinical Trial requires compliance of ethical requirements.
- Re-challenge for scientific interest is not appropriate but can be done if it offers clinical benefit to the patients.

Bibliography

1. Contemporary Ethical Issues in Biomedical and Health Research, Indian Council of Medical Research, August 2007.
2. A Practical Handbook on the Pharmacovigilance of Antiretroviral Medicines, World Health Organization, 2009.
3. Current Challenges in Pharmacovigilance: Pragmatic Approaches, Report of CIOMS Working Group V, Geneva, 2001.

Chapter 11

Global Scenario in Pharmacovigilance

"Doctors are men who prescribe medicines of which they know little, to cure diseases of which they know less, in human beings of who they nothing".

Voltaire

After reading this chapter, you should be able to understand and appreciate:
• The Role and Contribution of International Agencies – WHO, ICH and CIOMS;
• The Pharmacovigilance Systems of other Countries – Australia, UK, and USA.

The medicines are used throughout the globe and so are the incidences of adverse events. No medicine is safe all the time for all persons. The occurrence of adverse drug reaction varies from one geographical region to the other due to several factors including the formulation of medicines (locally manufactured), customs and diets, and genetic variations. There are Pharmacovigilance programmes throughout the globe but intensity or extent of programme varies based on economic situation. The rich and industrial countries have robust programme and the poor and developing countries may not have that robust but a programme in one or other form. The international agencies like World Health Organization (WHO), International Conference on Harmonization (ICH) and Council for International Organizations of Medical Sciences (CIOMS) have been significantly contributing in promoting Pharmacovigilance activities in an attempt to improve patient safety through safe medications.

World Health Organization

World Health Organization, a specialized health agency of United Nations (but not subordinate to UN), started functioning on 7th April 1948 with an objective "the attainment by all peoples' of highest level of health". This 7th April, day of adoption of WHO's constitution, is celebrated as World Health Day every year. It has the mandate to develop, establish and promote international standards (on safety, purity and potency) with respect to food, biological and pharmaceutical and similar products.

The thalidomide disaster in 1961 (details can be seen elsewhere in the book) raised international concern on unsafe medications. A Resolution (WHA16.36) of Sixteenth World Health Assembly in 1963 re-affirming the need for early action in regard to rapid dissemination of information on adverse drug reaction led to the creation of the WHO Pilot Research Project for International Drug Monitoring in 1968. The purpose of the project was to develop an internationally acceptable system for detecting previously unknown or poorly understood adverse effects of medicines.

The Pilot Research Project for International Drug Monitoring of 1968 is now grown into a full- fledged WHO programme and is currently coordinated by the Uppsala Monitoring Centre. The Essential Medicines and Health Products (EMP) division of Health Systems and Innovations (HIS) cluster is responsible for the pharmacovigilance activities. WHO programme began just with ten countries contributing to the international database in 1968 and now 120 countries contributing. India joined the WHO programme in 1998. The WHO database is now enriched with more than 10 million case reports which testify the success story of WHO programme. The programme has brought together all the countries with one common vision of preventing patient harm.

The WHO has one more collaborating centre: the Netherlands Pharmacovigilance Centre Lareb as WHO Collaborating Centre for Pharmacovigilance in Education and Patient Reporting.

The WHO has published several booklets and documents which are useful in sensitizing and promoting pharmacovigilance activities. The WHO Pharmaceuticals Newsletter and WHO Drug Information are important publications through which WHO disseminate safety information. The WHO programme has developed a standardized adverse reaction terminology (WHO ART) and a comprehensive index of reported drugs (WHO DD). The WHO Drug Dictionary is unique in its coverage of drugs marketed throughout the world.

Open Access to Drug Safety Database: The World Health Organization has recently launched a new open access drug safety database called VigiAccess. VigiAccess is a new web based application that allows everyone to access information on reported cases of adverse events related to over 1,50,000 medicine and vaccines. More than 10 million cases reported from various countries to the WHO database can be accessed now at: www.vigiaccess.org.

Uppsala monitoring centre: The UMC is an independent foundation and a centre for international services and scientific research. Its priorities are the safety of the patients and safe and effective use of medicines in every part of the world.

The UMC has been carrying out the WHO's international drug monitoring activities since 1978. As a collaborating centre, it adheres to the WHO policies and works in close association with WHO headquarter. But organizationally and professionally it is distinct from WHO. It focuses on early detection of potential issues relating to use and safety of medicines. The main activities of UMC on pharmacovigilance are:

- Screening and analysing international adverse reaction data;
- Supporting effective communication of the most focused, up-to-date scientific information;
- Providing tools for data entry, management, retrieval, reference and research;
- Alerting regulating authorities of member countries about potential drug safety issues; and
- Capacity building through education and training in setting up and running national pharmacovigilance programmes as well as in using the UMC Tools.

The UMC has developed and uses several software tools to help the participating National Centres in international drug monitoring programme. These include VigiFlow, VigiBase, VigiMine, VigiMed, VigiSearch and VigiLyze.

Vigi flow: This is a simple web based individual case safety report (ICSR) management system that improves all aspects of ADR reporting. ICSR data can be manually entered into VigiFlow. Once a report is complete and committed the first version of the ICSR is generated and automatically saved in in global database called VigiBase. It is possible to retrieve reports for amendment or follow up.

Vigi base: This is the WHO's global ICSR database consisting of all reports received from member countries since 1968. This computerized database has information recorded in a structured and hierarchical form to allow for easy and flexible retrieval and analysis of data.

Vigi mine: It provides access to statistical data on all drug – ADR pairs available in VigiBase. VigiMine allows filtering of the results on a number of statistical criteria and stratification by age, sex, country and year of reporting. It reflects the statistical changes too.

Vigi med: This is a web based forum for people working in National Centres of WHO programme to have easy access to safety concerns in other countries, to check regulatory status and to expedite the sharing of drug information.

Vigi search: This is a search tool that provides access to all case reports in VigiBase and searching across multiple drugs and ADRs simultaneously even using a lot of filters. The data can be accessed on an overview level and viewed from number of aspects including individual case report.

Vigi lyze: This is a powerful search and analysis tool that provides access to VigiBase. It can be used to have global, regional or national view of an identified ADR and monitor international patient safety data. It offers international comparison with national spontaneous reporting data and provides access to ADR information of drugs which are not yet available for use in national market. The unique feature of this tool is that the results are instantly available both in tabular and graphic forms.

Each member state collects, processes and evaluates adverse drug reaction reports and submits the information to the WHO database. Case reports submitted on agreed format to the WHO VigiBase are checked for technical correctness and incorporated into the international database. They are screened periodically for new and serious reaction/s. The flow of information from national centres to the WHO database is described graphically.

International Conference on Harmonization (ICH): The International Conference on Harmonization of Technical Requirements for Registration of Pharmaceuticals for Human Use (ICH) is not a conference but an organization that provides platform for regulatory authorities and pharmaceutical industries of European Union, USA and Japan to design common guidelines for the development and registration of medicines. Though the guidelines are meant for these three regions but these regions have maximum consumption of medicines. Hence, the other countries are also interested on ICH guidelines as marketing of medicinal products becoming global. India too exports medicines to more than 200 countries including USA, UK, and Japan.

ICH was established in April 1990 and since then it has developed several guidelines, through consultative process, on Quality, Safety, Efficacy and Multidisciplinary. The pharmacovigilance guidelines are developed under safety guidelines. The safety guidelines cover the requirements of pre-clinical testing. The pharmacovigilance guidelines are:

- E2A – Clinical Safety Data Management [Definitions and Standards for Expedited Reporting]
- E2B(R3) – Clinical Safety Data Management [Data Elements for Transmission of Individual Case Safety Reports]
- E2B(R3) – Implementation [Electronic Transmission of Individual Case Safety Reports]
- E2C(R2) – Periodic Benefit : Risk Evaluation Report
- E2D – Post Approval Safety Data Management [Definitions and Standards for Expedited Reporting]
- E2E – Pharmacovigilance Planning
- E2F – Development Safety Update Report

Council for International Organizations of Medical Sciences (CIOMS): The CIOMS is an international not for profit organization established by WHO and United Nations Educational, Scientific and Cultural Organization (UNESCO) in 1949. It facilitates and promotes international activities in the field of biomedical sciences. In addition to other areas of works, the CIOMS has initiated activities on 'safety requirements for use of drugs' and 'assessment of and monitoring of adverse drug reactions and pharmacogenetics'. Through its working groups, CIOMS developed recommendations or guidance in the area of international reporting of adverse drug reactions including introduction of standardized reporting form [Copy is enclosed in the Appendix], international reporting of periodic drug safety update reports, core clinical safety information on drugs, evaluation of benefit/risk balance, current challenges of Pharmacovigilance, management of safety information from clinical trials, development safety update reports and signal detection in pharmacovigilance. These guidance documents are very helpful for all stake holders from industry to regulatory agencies.

Many of the recommendations of CIOMS are adopted by ICH. This has contributed significant impact on international drug regulation.

Pharmacovigilance in United Kingdom: Like several other countries the United Kingdom too initiated the systematic way of monitoring of adverse drug reactions soon after the outbreak of thalidomide disaster in 1960s. The Commission on Human Medicines (COHM) of Medicines and Healthcare Products Regulatory Agency (MHRA), an executive agency of Department of Health, is responsible for Pharmacovigilance activities.

The Committee on Safety of Drugs (CSD) of UK headed by Sir Derrick Dunlop had introduced the spontaneous reporting scheme in 1964 asking the members of the medical and dental profession to promptly report the details of any untoward condition in a patient which might be the result of drug treatment. It was known as 'Yellow Card System'. Now too it is known by the same name though pharmacovigilance has no association with yellow colour. The important features of the scheme were:

- Suspected adverse reactions should be reported;
- It was the responsibility of the doctor or dentist to submit report;
- There should not be delay in reporting; and
- Report and reporter's confidentiality was promised.

With the establishment of Licensing Authority in 1971, the Committee on Safety of Drugs was absorbed into it and new Committee was evolved as 'Committee on Safety of Medicines' (CSM). The terminology 'Drug' was thought to be too emotive and hence replaced with 'Medicine'.

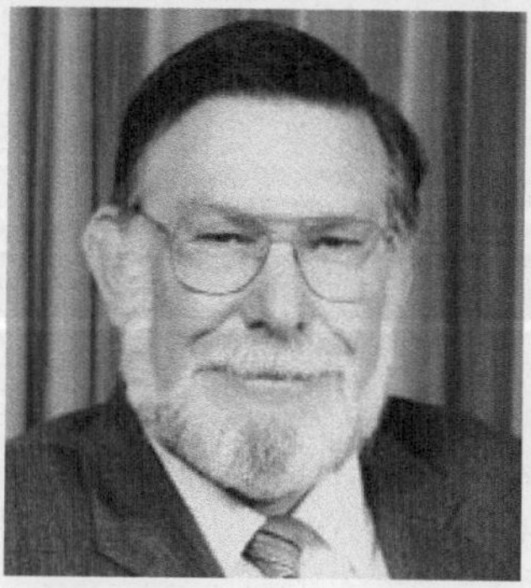

Professor William Inman, a polio affected doctor confined to wheel chair, is credited for developing Yellow Card System in UK for voluntary reporting of Adverse Drug Reaction. His study linking contraceptive pill with thrombosis led to the reduced dose of hormone without reducing the efficacy. This earned him the accolade "Father of the mini pill". He was the first to use the term Post Marketing Surveillance (PMS). Realizing the limitation of spontaneous reporting, he introduced another system for the Prescription Event Monitoring.

There have been several changes in the design of Yellow Card reporting form as the programme expanded. Initially it was the doctors or dentists who were authorized to submit the reports, now it is open to all healthcare professionals including nurses and pharmacists to patients. While for some countries like France, Norway, Sweden, and Spain, reporting of adverse drug reactions are compulsory; in UK it is voluntary. In order to promote reporting, the yellow cards are made available as a part of British National Formulary (BNF) and prescription pads.

The voluntary reporting forms are accepted by MHRA/COHM from both healthcare professionals and members of public. Reports are also received from marketing authorization holders [It is compulsory]. For established products, the MHRA requires that the healthcare professionals report only serious suspected adverse drug reactions. For new products, MHRA encourages the reporting of all suspected adverse reactions. Special attention is given on ADRs in children and elderly and on herbal medicines. Though data is obtained from wide sources, spontaneous reporting system is the main source for pharmacovigilance activities.

Orange Card Reporting: Orange card reporting is a separate initiative of MHRA in collaboration with British Paediatric Surveillance Unit (BPSU) (now known as Royal College of Paediatrics and Child Health) where consultant paediatricians are encouraged to report particular disorders under surveillance in children to the BPSU.

MHRA has ADR online information tracking (ADROIT) database. The reports are entered to ADROIT and MHRA evaluates them to assess the causal relationship between the drugs and reported reactions. Then agency identifies the possible risk factors. The marketing authorization holders have access to ADROIT and there are provisions of exchange of pharmacovigilance data electronically. The MHRA communicates the regulatory decisions through circulation of 'Current Problems in Pharmacovigilance Bulletin' to doctors and pharmacists. In order to disseminate urgent hazard warning "Dear Healthcare Professionals" letters are sent by post and electronically. The fact sheets and safety alerts are placed in website too.

UK was one of the founding members of WHO programme on International Drug Monitoring. Being a member of the European Union, the PV guidance of EU is applicable in UK.

United States of America

The US FDA is responsible for safety monitoring of medicines and it continues to assess the benefit–risk profile throughout the life cycle of the product. The primary purpose of the pharmacovigilance is the generation of signals or hypothesis of a potential adverse drug effect association. USFDA safety information and adverse event reporting programme is known as MedWatch.

Database: The safety signals may arise from different sources, but the most common is the voluntary or spontaneous case reporting to the regional or National pharmacovigilance centres or FDA. The healthcare professionals or patients voluntarily send the ADR case reports either to manufacturer or to FDA. The report received by FDA either from healthcare professionals, patients or manufacturers are entered into FDA Adverse Event Reporting System (FAERS). *The significant feature is that the database, FAERS, contains not just the ADR reports but also reports on medication errors. The modern pharmacovigilance includes the medication error within its domain.* FAERS is the repository of ADR and medication error.

Report submission: Individual reporter like health professionals (physicians, pharmacists, nurses, and others) or consumers (patients, family members, lawyers and others) can directly submit the adverse event reports to the USFDA. This is voluntary. The manufacturers have the mandatory obligation to submit the reports: A serious ADR is to be submitted within 15 days of the receipt of the report. For most non-prescription products manufacturers are not required to submit the ADR reports to FDA. The format for submitting the report is available in MedWatch website. For the interest of the readers it is kept in appendix. The electronic submission system is also practiced.

Processing of reports: Serious unlabelled ADR reports submitted by manufacturers, Serious ADR reports (labeled or unlabelled) submitted directly to the FDA by healthcare professionals or consumers and reports of selected important medical events are evaluated by clinical reviewers in the Centre for Drug Evaluation and Research (CDER) and the Centre for Biologics Evaluation and Research (CBER). If potential safety concern is identified in FAERS, further evaluation is performed. Then further investigation including computer search of entire database of adverse event reports, literature review, drug usage data and incidence rate are done.

An analysis of the safety issue is then presented to the medical reviewing division responsible for ongoing regulation of the drug. If the signal is strong enough, the regulatory decision such as labeling changes, restricting the use of drug, communicating new safety information to the public and withdrawal from the market is initiated by the FDA.

The MedWatch uses e-mail communication to disseminate new safety information to the healthcare professionals. MedWatch receives reports of serious adverse events for all medical products except vaccines. The vaccine safety monitoring programme is known as "Post Licensure Rapid Immunization Safety Monitoring (PRISM)" Programme.

Australia: The Office of Medicine Safety Monitoring (OMSM), a branch of Therapeutic Good Administration (TGA) is the responsible authority for safety monitoring of medicines in Australia. TGA is the medicine regulatory authority and is a unit of Australian Government Department of Health and Aging (under Therapeutic Goods Act 1989). TGA has established pharmacovigilance system for the collection and evaluation of information relevant to the benefit to risk balance of registered medicinal products.

Each sponsor or manufacturer of registered medicine must have appropriate pharmacovigilance system in place in order to assure responsibility and liability for its product in the market and to assure that appropriate action can be taken when necessary. The company should have a medically qualified person responsible for pharmacovigilance. The separate sponsor may have same qualified person.

Report submission: The spontaneous adverse event reporting is voluntary in Australia. The healthcare professionals, patients and consumers may report to the sponsors or manufacturers or directly to TGA through Adverse Drug Reaction Advisory Committee (ADRAC) using "Blue Card". The report can be submitted by post to The Secretary, ADRAC, and no postage is necessary if posted in Australia.

ADRAC was formed in 1970 to advise TGA on safety of medicines.

All serious adverse drug reaction reports whether expected or unexpected received by sponsor from healthcare professionals, patients, and consumers are to be reported to ADRAC in an expedited manner [within 15 calendar days]. Cases from worldwide literature review and reports from post-registration studies are also to be reported within 15 days of receipt.

Sponsors are not required to submit the serious reports of foreign origin on an expedited basis. On the other hand, sponsors are required to advise the TGA within 72 hours of any significant safety issue identified as a result of ongoing review process or action taken by foreign regulatory authority. Significant safety issue means withdrawal or suspension of availability of the product; additional information like contraindication added to an approved drug; and modification of alert.

The non-serious ADR reports should be submitted only on request from TGA or included in PSUR.

Web based reporting system is available.

Pharmacovigilance Requirement for Sponsor of Registered and Listed Medicines

Report Type	Method / Format of Report	Reporting Time Limit
Serious adverse reaction	Blue Card / CIOMS Form / Online Reporting Form	Within 15 calendar days
Significant safety issue	In writing to post-marketing surveillance branch by facsimile or e. mail	Within 72 hours of receipt
Non-serious adverse events	In requested format	As PSUR or as asked by TGA

The sponsor is required to submit PSUR annually for the first three years after the date of approval letter. The first report must be submitted not later than 15 calendar months after approval. The subsequent report must be submitted at least annually from the date of submission of first report.

Processing of reports: TGA's Office of Medicine Safety Monitoring receives reports of suspected adverse events associated with prescription medicines, vaccines, OTC medicines and complementary medicines. On receipt of reports, they are reviewed by professional staff. Reports involving serious reactions or recently marketed drugs are reviewed by adverse drug reaction committee, a sub-committee of Australian Drug Evaluation Committee (ADEC).

After the medical review, if any new safety information is required to be disseminated, the new safety information is circulated to the healthcare professionals through Australian ADRAC bulletin.

Australia participates in International Drug Monitoring Programme managed by Uppsala Centre.

Key Messages

- WHO Programme for International Drug Monitoring was started as a pilot research project in 1968.
- WHO Programme is now coordinated by the Uppsala Monitoring Centre (UMC) in Sweden. The UMC is the WHO collaborating centre for international drug monitoring. 120 countries are currently contributing to the WHO database.
- The Netherlands Pharmacovigilance Centre Lareb is the WHO collaborating centre for pharmacovigilance in education and patient reporting.
- UMC developed several information technology based tools to help the participating national centres: VigiFlow, VigiBase, VigiMine, VigiMed, VigiSearch and VigiLyze.
- CIOMS, an associate of WHO, offers a forum for policy makers, pharmaceutical industries, government agencies and academics to make recommendation on the communication of safety information between regulators and pharmaceutical industries.
- ICH, a platform of drug regulation authorities and pharmaceutical industries of European Union, USA and Japan, has several guidelines on quality, safety and efficacy and multidisciplinary guidance on harmonizing the requirements for registration of medicines for human use. The pharmacovigilance guidelines come under efficacy guidance.
- In UK, the pharmacovigilance activities are managed by Commission on Human Medicine under MHRA. The programme is dependent on voluntary reporting of suspected adverse drug reactions by healthcare professionals and the members of public. The programme is called Yellow Card System. UK was one of the founding members of WHO programme on International Drug Monitoring.
- In USA, FDA is the regulatory authority for safety monitoring of drugs and other medicinal products including medical devices and vaccines. The adverse event monitoring of products other than vaccines are managed through MedWatch. The US programme includes medication error too in pharmacovigilance domain. The adverse events data base is called FAERS. For healthcare professionals and consumers, reporting to FDA is voluntary while for manufacturers it is mandatory.
- Office of Medicine Safety Monitoring of Therapeutic Goods Administration is the agency responsible for pharmacovigilance (safety monitoring) activities in Australia. It is necessary that the sponsor must have appropriate pharmacovigilance system with qualified person being responsible. Spontaneous reporting by the healthcare professionals and patients is voluntary and is managed through Blue Card System. Sponsor is required to submit serious adverse event reports within 15 calendar days. It is not mandatory to submit the non-serious adverse events in expedited way but as PSUR.

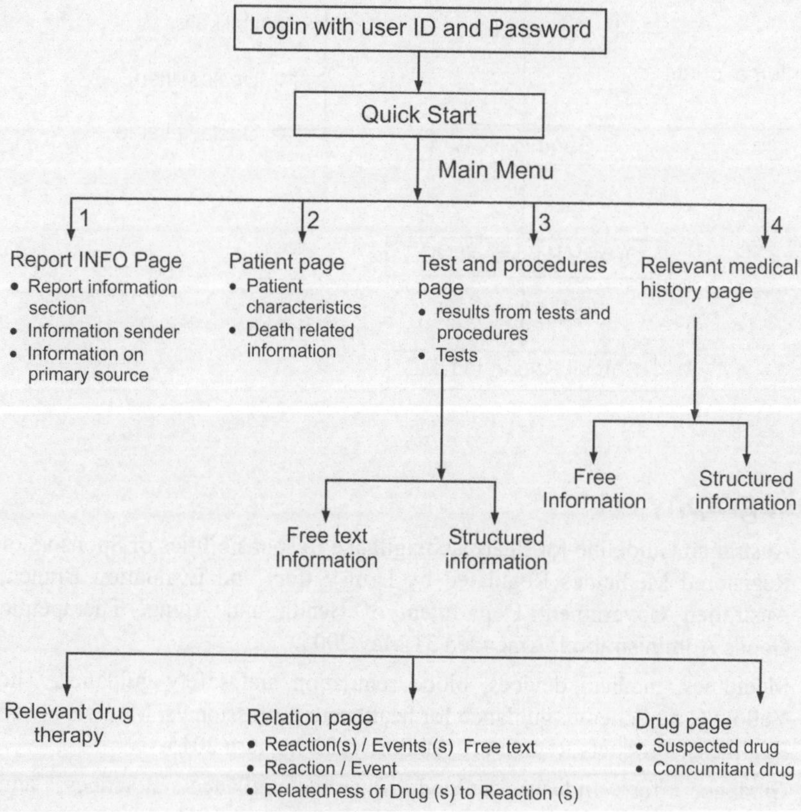
Login with user ID and Password
Quick Start
Main Menu
1
Report INFO Page
• Report information section
• Information sender
• Information on primary source
2
Patient page
• Patient characteristics
• Death related information
3
Test and procedures page
• results from tests and procedures
• Tests
4
Relevant medical history page
Free Information
Structured information
Free text Information
Structured information
Relevant drug therapy
Relation page
• Reaction(s) / Events (s) Free text
• Reaction / Event
• Relatedness of Drug (s) to Reaction (s)
Drug page
• Suspected drug
• Concumitant drug

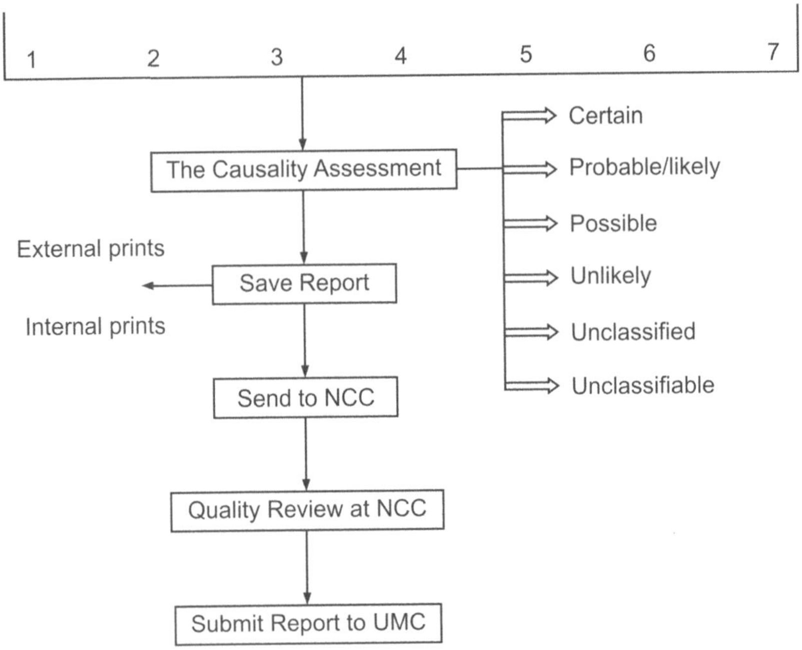

Bibliography

1. Australian Guideline for Pharmacovigilance Responsibilities of Sponsors of Registered Medicines Regulated by Drug Safety and Evaluation Branch, Australian Government Department of Health and Aging, Therapeutic Goods Administration, Amended 31 May 2005.
2. Medicines, medical devices, blood regulation and safety guidance, The Yellow Card Scheme: guidance for healthcare professionals, Medicines and Healthcare Products Regulatory Authority, 23 January 2015.
3. Guidance for Industry, Good Pharmacovigilance Practices and Pharmacoepidemiologic Assessment, US Department of Health and Human Services, FDA, March 2005.
4. Ronald D. Mann and Elizabeth B. Andrews (Editors), Pharmacovigilance, Second Edition, John Wiley and Sons, Ltd., 2007.
5. http://www.who-umc.org accessed on 25 March 2015.

Chapter 12

Pharmacovigilance of Ayurveda, Siddha and Unani Medicines

All substances are poisonous, there is none which is not a poison; the right dose differentiates a poison from a remedy.

Paracelsus

After reading this chapter, you should be able to understand and appreciate:
• The basic philosophies of Ayurveda, Siddha and Unani (ASU) Medicines.
• The need of Pharmacovigilance of Indian Systems of Medicines.
• Salient points of National Pharmacovigilance Programmes of ASU Medicines.
• Challenges of Safety Surveillance of ASU Medicines.

In spite of tremendous developments in the field of modern medicines, the people of India still have limited access to them. A large section of the population continue to rely on the Indian Systems of Medicine (ISM) for their health care for many reasons such as easy availability and affordability. People too believe that they are from natural source and thus are safer compared to modern medicines. Indian Systems of Medicine, a conglomerate of Ayurveda, Siddha and Unani (ASU), has a long history. The popular belief that the medicines of natural origin are harmless and free from side effects is not true. Various studies have shown the serious issues with respect to herbs' safety. The presence of toxic materials in the ASU medicines are reported in reputed scientific journals. The detection of heavy metals in these products further causes safety concern. The presence of heavy metals in medicinal products at a concentration beyond the acceptable limit can cause serious health hazards including kidney failure.

Ayurveda, aptly known as 'Science of Life', is an ancient Indian healthcare system and its history can be traced back to 2500 BC or so. The distinguished feature of Ayurveda is the holistic nature with which it considers a human being in totality and takes into consideration his relationship with the environment. It is known for its comprehensive approach involving life style modulation, biopurification therapy and use of palliative remedies and avoidance of factors that are predisposing or precipitating for disease genesis. Accordingly to Ayurveda, the whole world as well as the human beings are made up of five basic elements *[Earth (Prithvi); Water (Jal); Fire (Agni); Air (Vayu) and Ether (Akasha)]* and are governed by three *doshas* (humours): *Vata, Pitta* and *Kapha.* The balanced state three *doshas* maintains the body functions and the imbalance causes diseases. Ayurveda aims counteracting these imbalances of three *doshas.* The Ayurvedic medicines are of plant, animal and or mineral origin and use both single drug or compounded formulations. There are two basic safety issues: inherent presence of toxic substances in the product and unacceptable level of impurities such as microbial contaminants, pesticides, residual solvents and heavy metals. The Drugs and Cosmetics Act of the country has recognized the use of toxic substances in the preparation of Ayurvedic medicines. These substances are listed in Schedule E1 of the Drugs and Cosmetics Rules. During the preparation of medicinal products containing such substances, there is a need to undertake detoxication (called shodhan) as mentioned in authoritative ancient texts. Ayurvedic formulations containing poisonous substances, metals, etc. if not used according to Ayurvedic principles may show symptoms of toxicity. Ayurvedic experts outline the following factors responsible for toxicity of Ayurvedic medicines:

- ***Improper manufacturing process:*** The authoritative ancient Ayurvedic texts describe the methods of detoxication of metals used in Ayurveda. When the relevant procedure is not followed but a short cut way is accepted for manufacturing, it can lead to toxicity;
- ***Presence of contaminants:*** The heavy metals are often added deliberately. There is no control over this especially when they are prepared by individuals. One study showed that 17 out of 70 Ayurvedic products tested had heavy metals [Journal of American Medical Association, 2004, 292 (23), 2868-73]. Other studies showed the presence of allopathic drugs like phenytoin

and Phenobarbital in Ayurvedic medicines meant for epilepsy treatment and presence of corticosteroids in many Ayurvedic medicines.

- ***Improper use:*** The Ayurvedic medicines are to be used with respect to the vehicle (honey, water etc), relationship with the food (early morning empty stomach, immediately before food, immediately after food, etc.) and dose etc. If the procedure is not adhered to, it may lead to toxicity.
- ***Poor quality:*** Ensuring consistent uniform quality of Ayurvedic medicines is often difficult as the raw materials quality varies widely from source to source and even from the same source at different seasons. The microbial contamination and toxicity of residual solvents used in extraction too cause toxicity to the products.

A married couple showed elevated blood lead levels after taking Ayurvedic herbal medicines, dispensed from an Indian hospital. The male, who had taken the unidentified Ayurvedic medicine for five months was admitted to a hospital in Australia with abdominal pain, nausea and vomiting secondary to lead poisoning. He had a lead level of 120 μg/dL and also high levels of arsenic and mercury. His wife was asymptomatic but also had a high lead level of 40 μg/dL. An acceptable blood concentration for lead is < 10 μg/dL.

The Drugs Regulatory of Australia has released a statement about the safety of Ayurvedic medicines in Australia, in response to recent research into the toxic content of heavy metals found in some Ayurvedic medicines.

There are several possible explanations for the presence of heavy metals in traditional herbal remedies. Salts of heavy metals (for example those of lead, mercury and arsenic) are used as principal ingredients in some traditional Indian and to a lesser extent in Chinese herbal remedies. In addition, cross-contamination of ingredients can occur between these types of products and products not intended to contain metal salts if manufacturing conditions are not controlled.

Australian Adverse Drug Reaction Bulletin, Vol 26, No. 1, February 2007.

The argument that the Ayurvedic medicines have been in use for thousands of years and there have been very little reports of side effects. This should be the enough evidence of safety of Ayurvedic medicines. The Ayurvedic medicines are no longer prepared or manufactured based on the procedure outlined in the ancient texts but the modern technology. The modernized Ayurvedic medicines cannot be treated on par with the medicines described in ancient authoritative Ayurvedic texts. Safety monitoring of these modern Ayurvedic medicines is a necessity not only in the interest of Ayurveda but also in larger public interest.

Siddha Medicines are of Dravidian origin and is mostly practiced in Tamil Nadu. According to Siddha medicines, there are seven elements: *Saram (plasma), Cheneer (blood), Ooun (muscle), Kozhuppu (fat), Elumbu (bone), Moolai (nerve),* and *Sukila* or *Inthiriyam (semen)* that are responsible for physical, physiological and psychological functions of the human body. These seven elements are activated by three components or humors: *Vatha (air), Pitha (fire* or *heat* or *energy)* and *Kapha (water).* It is believed that these humors are in a particular ratio in human body and disturbance of this equilibrium causes illness. Diet, physical activities and environmental conditions are the main cause for disturbance of the humor equilibrium. Most of the Siddha medicines are based on Herbo-minerals and metallic, which are more effective than the single and compound herbal drug preparations. In short, the basic concept of Siddha Medicine is similar to Ayurveda but the mode of preparation is different.

Unani Medicines owe their origin to Greece and the foundation of the system is based on the teaching of Hippocrates, the father modern medicine. Arabs introduced the system to India. The system is based on humoral theory which believes the presence of four humors: *Dam (blood), Balghum (phlegm), Safra (yellow bile),* and *Sauda (black bile).* There is unique humoral constitution in every person representing his/her health status. The body has the power of self preservation or adjustment. The weakening of this power causes imbalance in the humoral composition and causes disease. The medicines help the body to regain this power and restore the humoral balance. The correct diet and digestion are very important to the system. The medicines are mostly of herbal origin though some medicines may be with animal and mineral origin.

National pharmacovigilance programme for ayurveda, siddha and unani medicines: On the similar lines of National Pharmacovigilance Programme for modern medicines, the National Programme for ASU medicines was initiated with the assistance of World Health Organization Country Office for India. The Institute for Post Graduate Teaching & Research in Ayurveda, Gujarat Ayurveda University, had taken the lead in developing the protocol for the National Programme. The programme is funded by the Department of AYUSH, Ministry of Health and Family Welfare, Government of India [Now AYUSH has separate independent Ministry].

The salient points of the programme are:

- The objectives of the programme are classified as: Short term objective – to develop the culture of notification, Medium term objective – to involve healthcare professionals and professional associations in the drug monitoring and information dissemination processes, and Long term objective – to achieve operational efficiencies that would make National Programme a bench mark for global drug monitoring.
- A three tier system is identified: National Pharmacovigilance Resource Centre – One; Regional Pharmacovigilance Centres – Eight; and Peripheral Pharmacovigilance Centres – Thirty. Institute for Post Graduate Teaching & Research in Ayurveda, Gujarat Ayurveda University is appointed as National Pharmacovigilance Resource Centre.
- The programme advocates the reports of: all adverse reactions suspected to have caused by the ASU medicines alone or along with any other medicine; all suspected drug interactions; reactions to any other drug which are suspected of significantly affecting patient's management including reactions suspected of causing death, life threatening, hospitalization, disability, congenital anomaly or required intervention to prevent permanent impairment or damage.
- All registered medical practitioners of ASU systems and other paramedical persons involved in healthcare like nurses, pharmacists, primary health care workers etc. can report the suspected adverse drug event. The programme does not accept the report directly from the consumers or patients.
- The collected adverse drug reaction data are planned to be handed confidentially and statistical analysis of the data are to be forwarded to the Department of AYUSH, Government of India.

Challenges of the PV programme of ASU: While it is anticipated that data generated through the PV programme of ASU medicines would provide more confidence among the users and help in promoting global acceptability of ASU medicines, there are many challenges too. There is no regular budget to make the programme self-sustainable. It is necessary to earmark the budget for continuity of the programme. More awareness and training programme is to be conducted at various levels to sensitise the ASU health professionals on the importance of Pharmacovigilance and benefits of their reporting. Many times, the consumers do take these medicines at their wish considering that they do have no side effects. The consumers even fail or do not think it necessary to tell the physicians about their self medication. Under such circumstances, it is often difficult to assign the reasons for identified adverse drug reactions. As the products composition often varies from manufacturer to manufacturer and sometimes not labelled, it becomes more difficult to identify the suspected drug.

There is no appropriate medicine classification [the anatomical – therapeutic – chemical (ATC)] for all ASU medicines and it provides a big challenges coding ASU medicines for international comparison.

Global resurgence of Ayurveda especially its herbal component necessitates the need of its scientific validation in terms of safety and efficacy. The National PV Programme of ASU drugs has to go a long way establishing the scientific evidence of safety of ISM. Now, with AYUSH as a separate ministry, it is expected that the programme would receive greater attention in public interest as well as in popularising ISM globally.

Key Messages

- Ayurvedic (Vedic origin), Siddha (Dravidian origin) and Unani (Greek origin) have long history of use in India. They are either herbal or herbo-mineral products.
- The popular believe that herbs or natural means safe is not true. There are two basic safety issues: inherent presence of toxic substances in the product and unacceptable level of microbial counts, pesticides, residual solvents and heavy metals.
- The safety issues of ASU medicines are reported in many scientific publications.
- The National Pharmacovigilance Programme for ASU medicines was initiated during 2008 with Institute for Post Graduate Teaching & Research in Ayurveda, Gujarat Ayurveda University, as National Resource Centre.
- There are several constraints in promoting pharmacovigilance activities of ASU medicines. These include no regular budgetary support, ignorance of consumers and ASU professionals on safety issues, product variation from manufacturer to manufacturer and lack of appropriate classification of medicines.

Bibliography

1. WHO guidelines on safety monitoring of herbal medicines in pharmacovigilance systems, World Health Organization, Geneva, 2004.

2. Guidelines for the Regulation of Herbal Medicines in South East Asia Region, WHO – SEARO, 2004.
3. Ayurveda and its Scientific Aspects: Opportunities for Globalization, Department of AYUSH and Council of Scientific and Industrial Research, Government of India, 2006.
4. National Pharmacovigilance Protocol for Ayurveda, Siddha and Unani (ASU) Drugs, National Pharmacovigilance Resource Centre, Gujarat Ayurveda University, 2008.
5. Galib and Rabinarayan Acharya, National P Pharmacovigilance Programme for Ayurveda, Siddha and Unani Drugs, AYU, 29 (4), 2008.
6. Syed Zia-ur Rahman, Rahat Ali Khan and Abdul Latif, Pharmacovigilance in Unani Medicine – A Challenge, The Pharma Review, July – August, 2011.

Chapter 13

Case Studies on Drugs Withdrawal

"If you look over a list of medicinal recipe in vogue in the last century, how foolish and useless they are seem to be! And yet we use equally absurd ones with faith today".

Henry David Thoreau

Thalidomide: the Greatest Drug Disaster

Thalidomide is perhaps one of the greatest drug tragedies that has changed the course of safety monitoring (Pharmacovigilance) system in the world. The drug was synthesized in 1956 by a German company, Chemie. The invention of thalidomide was a new venture for the company which used to make cosmetics and household products. The company had little or no experience on pharmaceuticals. Thalidomide showed considerable promise as a sleeping tablet and as an alternative to barbiturate. It had better safety profile than barbiturate as overdosing 100 times the normal dose was not lethal. Besides, it did not have the risk of 'hangover' effects that might affect driving or operating heavy machineries.

The company started marketing thalidomide in Germany in October 1957 under the name of Contergan. Its equivalent Distaval was marketed in England. It was hailed as "tranquiliser of the future". Within a year of thalidomide's introduction in Germany, an extremely rare birth deformity began to appear. Babies were born with short, finlike flaps instead of normal arms and legs. It was in November 1961, a German paediatrician declared that the outbreak of this gross malformation, phocomelia, to the use in the pregnancy of the new hypnotic drug. In 1961 December, the first report of association was published in a widely circulated medical journal indicating that thalidomide might be human teratogen. The number of cases of phocomelia had mysteriously increased from 12 in 1959, to 83 in 1960, to 360 in 1961 in Germany alone. It was estimated that more than 10,000 babies of twenty countries were the victim of thalidomide. Of these, around 50% (5000) survived and 1600 of whom eventually needed artificial limbs. The drug was finally withdrawn in 1961.

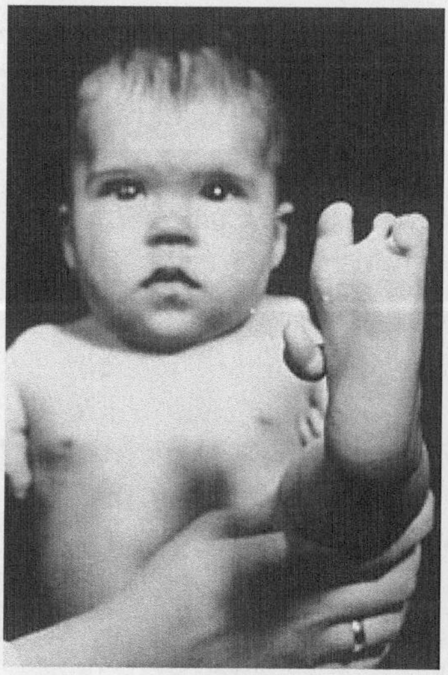

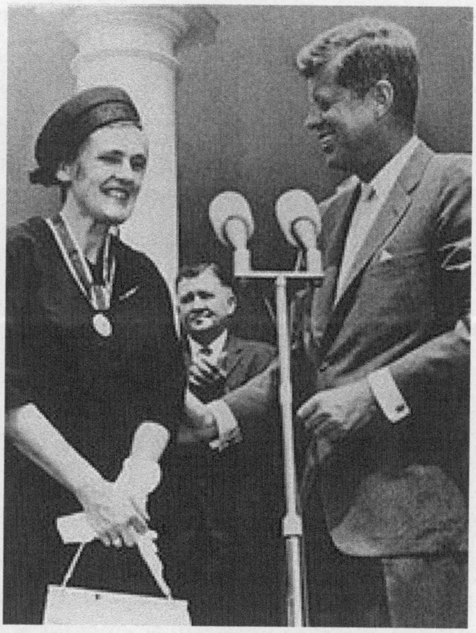

In 1960, a US pharmaceutical company, Merrell Pharmaceuticals, applied for permission to market in USA. By this time many countries had permitted its use. In October 1961, the newly joined medical officer, Dr. (Ms.) Frances Kelsey, was assigned the task of supervising the approval process of thalidomide. At that time, USFDA had to reject the approval within 60 days or automatically allow marketing. Though the company was eagerly waiting for its approval, Kelsey kept on stalling after each 60 days period rejecting the application incomplete. She was apprehensive of some data: one of the side effects was mild neuritis or tingling of nerves. She was trying to correlate her research of fifteen years before that the neuritis of this type in pregnant animals resulted in deformed offspring. She was just waiting for little longer before making a decision which paid. Then of course, the non-lethal but shocking adverse effect of thalidomide was known to the world. While the children of more than 20 countries including UK, Australia, Belgium, Switzerland, were affected by this thalidomide, FDA medical officer, Kelsey saved the America by her heroic 'no' to thalidomide despite pressure. In 1962, Dr. Frances Kelsey was awarded the President's Gold Medal for distinguished service.

A review of the experimental work carried out with thalidomide before marketing revealed that inappropriate toxicological data had been published and animal findings were misinterpreted. Thalidomide disaster had taught many lessons and is also classic example to cite:

- A clear understanding of benefit and risk: No medicine is absolutely safe. It is the benefit: risk ratio that makes the usefulness of substance as medicine. Thalidomide has now made a comeback as drug for refractory multiple myeloma and leprosy. In these patients, it outweighs risk in favour of benefit, provided it is not given to fertile women.
- It is not that everyone is at the same risk of a particular adverse effect. Women who do not have child bearing capacity have no risk at all.

In spite of so much negative publicity of thalidomide, this appears to be still used for nausea and alleviating morning sickness. In a related case, one petitioner alleged that he suffers from the disorder which has affected two fingers each on both his hands due to thalidomide prescription to mother. Bombay High Court has asked the Food and Drug Administration (FDA) to consider issuing a circular for doctors pointing out the side effects of the drug 'thalidomide'. [Source: http://drugscontrol.org/news.asp?id=8749&hl=Consider%20issuing%20circular%20on%20side-effects%20of%20drug:%20HC%20to%20FDA, accessed on 15 October 2013].

Bibliography

1. Mohanta, G. P., P. K. Manna, and R. Manavalan. "Drug Tragedies-A Review." Indian Journal of Pharmaceutical Education, 35.2 (2001): 65-66.
2. Charles F. Levinthal, Drugs, Behavior, and Modern Society, Second Edition, Allyn and Bacon, USA, 1999.
3. Bill Inman, Don't tell the patient, Highland Park Production, USA, 1999.

Diethylstilbestrol – Once a Popular Remedy only with Risk without Benefit!

The drug was promoted as a preventive measure for miscarriage based on the theory that habitual abortion was caused due to lack of progesterone and could be prevented by giving oestrogen that would in turn stimulate the production of progesterone. Based on this just theory, it was prescribed to millions of patients worldwide over 30 years and was stopped when it was found to cause cancer. This is diethylstilbestrol (DES). This was three times more potent than natural oestrogen. Though the use of DES has been discontinued since early 1970s, its impact on DES children continues! It has been described as a toxic time bomb referring to the long gestation period for the side effects to emerge and the effects may even stretch into third generations. The adverse effects was not only restricted to the user, the women during pregnancy, but has been percolated to the sons and daughters of the user.

DES, a first synthetic female hormone (oestrogen), was developed by Sir Edward Charles Dodds in 1938. He was a British Biochemist and was looking for synthetic oestrogens that could be easily and inexpensively made to treat symptoms of menopause. The beauty of DES was that it can be taken orally unlike the natural oestrogen and was not patented. The several pharmaceutical companies across the globe exploited this molecule and promoted for preventing abortion, miscarriage, premature labour and for several other conditions. In USA alone 267 pharmaceutical companies sold DES. A poorly designed study of 632 pregnant women reported in 1948 "the administration of DES could increase the chance of successful in women who had previous miscarriage or suffered from high blood pressure and risk of premature deliveries would be avoided". This has further promoted the prescription of DES.

The animal studies between 1930 and 1940 showed that DES and other oestrogens could cause cancer. The clinical studies proved its ineffectiveness. A randomised controlled trial involving 1600 women reported in 1953 showed that DES did not reduce the incidence of abortion, prematurity or post maturity. However, it was claimed that the investigators failed to report its adverse effects or risks from the study data. The study data showed significant increased abortion, neonatal deaths and premature births. Though animal studies showed the link between DES and cancer earlier, the link in humans was found only in 1971. The research showed a rare form of vaginal and cervical cancer in daughters of women who had taken DES early in pregnancy. It was found in the women in their early twenties. DES effect was termed as medically used disease. Following these reports, the US FDA in 1971 advised the physicians to discontinue prescribing DES to pregnant women. Other countries reacted slowly. Its use in pregnancy continued in France till 1977.

The DES was never banned but its indication in pregnancy was only withdrawn. Its use continued for the treatment of advanced prostate cancer, advanced breast cancer in post menopausal women, inhibition of lactation, amenorrhoea, vaginal irritation and morning after pill (post coital contraceptive). The use of DES in USA was continued till 1997. The DES was also promoted in veterinary practice as growth stimulant. People taking these animal foods were also exposed to the effects of DES. The DES is currently in use for the treatment of breast cancer and prostate cancer.

The DES was not only ineffective for the purpose for which it was promoted, it caused several adverse effects including impacting at least three generations. It had caused cell adenocarcinoma, a rare cancer in DES daughters (daughters of mothers taken DES during pregnancy). The risk is rare and range from one in 1000 to one in 10,000 exposed daughters. In addition, there were other risks: DES daughters were at twice risk to develop pre-cancerous abnormalities of the cervix, vagina and carcinoma in situ; development of adenosis (more abundant vaginal discharge); development of structural defects of cervix, vagina, uterus, fallopian tubes; more likely to be infertile; increased risk of adverse pregnancy outcomes; four time the risk of miscarriage and preterm labour; and the more chances of life threatening ectopic pregnancy. The DES sons too have their share of risk like increase in epididymal and testicular abnormalities such as undescended testes, incomplete or defective testicular developments and low sperm counts.

It has been estimated that a large number of women worldwide were exposed to action of DES: 20 to 30 lakh in USA, 40 lakh in Canada, 40 lakh in Europe, 2 lakh in France and 10 thousand in Australia. Realising the long term impact of DES use, the authorities advised the DES daughters to undergo annual cytological screening and colposcopic examination of both the cervix and vagina. The DES daughters of above 40 are advised annual mammography.

Many lawsuits have been filed in different parts of the world claiming compensation for the victims of DES. As there were large number of brands and considerable time is lapsed, it was difficult for the people to recollect the brand or company. In 1980, California Supreme Court ruled that the women should be able to fight as a group and the companies are liable to pay based on their market share. In a similar judgement in 1992, the Dutch Supreme Court ruled that every manufacturer should be equally and fully liable for damages, regardless of their market share at that time. In one judgement (2012) ordered 14 pharmaceutical companies to negotiate compensation for 53 women who alleged that their breast cancer was caused by their mothers' use of DES a decade ago. Perhaps the first settlement between four sisters and the Eli Lily has been reached in early 2013. It was alleged that the company did not test the drug adequately before marketing.

The use of DES though thought to be safe and effective, it was proved otherwise. The administration of any oestrogen is contraindicated during pregnancy. Its complete adverse effects are not yet known. As it is expected to harm even the third generation, we need to wait for the time when the youngest DES daughters reach the age of menopause perhaps by 2040. The DES is one of the greatest drug disasters but little focussed on its tragic effects.

Bibliography

1. Chetly, A., The time bomb explodes in Problem Drugs, Health Action International, 1993.
2. Diethylstilboestrol (DES) Exposure in Utero, College Statement of The Royal Australian and New Zealand College of Obstetricians and Gynaecologists, March 2013.
3. DES Update Home, http://www.cdc.gov/des/index.html accessed on 07 December 2013.
4. British National Formulary (63), March 2012.
5. Martindale: The Complete Drug Reference, Thirty fourth edition, Pharmaceutical Press, 2005.

Rofecoxib (Vioxx) – Association with Serious Cardiovascular Events

The harm caused by the use of Rofecoxib is regarded the single greatest drug safety catastrophe in USA and possibly in the history of the world. It was believed that this could have been largely or completely avoided. A senior US FDA officer testified that it might have caused more than 1, 00,000 heart attacks and strokes including an estimated 40,000 deaths. The drug was withdrawn by the innovator company in 2004 just after five years of use.

Rofecoxib was introduced in US market by Merck in 1999 with the brand name vioxx as an effective and safer alternative to NSAIDs for the treatment of pain associated with osteoarthritis. Rofecoxib is the selective cyclooxygenase -2 (COX-2) inhibitor. It was believed that selective inhibition of COX-2 enzyme would provide relief from pain and inflammation. As it does not interfere in COX-1, the production of COX-1 would remain and protect the gastrointestinal tract. The traditional NSAIDs provide relief from pain and inflammation through reducing the production of prostaglandin. Prostaglandins are produced at the site of injury and inflammation thus reduction of these provide anti-inflammatory effects. Prostaglandins do help protecting the stomach lining from acidic effect of gastric fluid. The traditional NSAIDs inhibit both the COX – 1 and COX – 2 enzymes and reduce the prostaglandin synthesis and thus provide anti-inflammatory effects and have long been associated with increased risk of gastrointestinal perforation, ulcers and bleeding. Thus the selective COX- 2 inhibitor, Rofecoxib, was termed as the miracle drug.

In reality the situation was different. The other effects of COX – 2 inhibitors were not given due importance in an attempt to conceal the safety data and promote Rofecoxib which was prescribed to more than 20 million Americans generating a revenue over USD 2 billion annually. The COX – 1 and the COX – 2 enzymes have different physiological roles. The COX – 1 produces thromboxane, a vasoconstrictor and platelet aggregator. On the other hand, COX – 2 enzyme produces prostacyclin, a vasodilator and anti-aggregating agent. Anti-aggregation of platelets and vasodilatation are important defence mechanisms for the human body when faced with onset of a cardiovascular event. Selective inhibition of COX – 2 enzyme disables this defence mechanism and the effects of COX – 1 thus puts the patients at higher risk of cardiovascular events.

The balance of COX – 1 and COX – 2 activities are disturbed. Besides, prostacyclin plays a role in the development of arteriosclerosis and in thinning of plaque along the wall of blood vessels. The particles of plaque are released due to rupture of the plaque and can cause thrombosis. This is the precise mechanism how the use of Rofecoxib was more risky in causing cardiovascular events.

Several studies reported the increased risk of cardiovascular events like increased heart attack with both low and high doses of rofecoxib use. There was even allegation that the Merck Company did know the risk but did not disclose. The company disseminated the pooled data of several small studies to promote the drug's cardiovascular safety to doctors in its cardio vascular card. The company's vioxx gastrointestinal outcomes research (VIGOR) launched in January 1999 was intended to expand the drug's approved indications comparing with naproxen for the treatment of rheumatoid arthritis. The authors withheld the critical data on cardiovascular toxicity. Its results were viewed with suspicion. Even though it was reported that the study did not follow Standard Operating Procedure (SOP), results disclosed in November 1999 showed 79% greater risk of deaths or cardiovascular events in one treatment group. A leading Medical Journal's Editor expressed that rofecoxib was not more effective than naproxen in relieving rheumatoid arthritis but did the halves the gastrointestinal risk. Another study called, APPROVe (Adenomatous Polyp Prevention on VIOXX) trial, was initiated to see if Vioxx 25 mg was effective in preventing the occurrence of colon polyps. Contrary to the expectation, the result showed an increased heart attacks and strokes after 18 months of continuous treatment compared to placebo. The study was stopped. In addition to its own research findings, the company came to know of the similar findings by USFDA, forced the Merck to withdraw its product Vioxx from the market effective 30 September 2004. There have been several legal suits. The company spent nearly $6bn as legal expense to settle vioxx related cases in USA alone. Many cases in UK and Australia too filed.

The funniest part was that its return to use was encouraged by USFDA with expanded safety warning and without advertising directly to the consumers. However, it did not return to the market. In India, the drug was manufactured and sold by several companies. The Government of India banned its use from 13 December 2004. A terrible tragedy could have been avoided had the company acted responsibly and the regulatory authority been more alert.

Bibliography

1. Harlan Krumholz *et al,* What have we learnt from Vioxx?, British Medical Journal, 334, 20 January 2007.
2. Janice Hopkins Tanne, Merck pays $ 1 bn penalty in relation to promotion of rofecoxib, British Medical Journal, 343, 28 November 2011.
3. Andy D. Birchfield, Jr *et al,* The Vioxx Story, a Portion of Plaintiff's position Paper in MDL# 1657, 2007.
4. Rofecoxib, Heart Attacks, and the FDA: Testimony of David J. Graham, November 18, 2004 (From The Revised A Lay person's Guide to Medicines, LOCOST, Vadodara, 2006).

Pioglitazone – Association with Bladder Cancer

The Government of India had suspended the manufacture, sale and distribution of popular anti-diabetic drug Pioglitazone in June 2013. But, it was subsequently reintroduced. The suspending notification claimed "the Government is satisfied that the use of drug Pioglitazone and all drug formulations containing Pioglitazone are likely to involve risk to human beings and the safer alternatives are available and hence the decision to suspend". The decision was not taken without following the standard procedure of discussion in DTAB (Drugs Technical Advisory Board) and without looking of hard evidence when the National Pharmacovigilance Programme is in place.

Pioglitazone belongs to the antidiabetic group of medicines 'thiazolidinediones (or glitazones)' was approved in US in early 1999. The two other drugs of the same glitazone group are withdrawn or severely restricted of use. Troglitazone within three years of introduction was removed because of its liver toxicity. Rosiglitazone is banned in many countries including India because of its association with elevated risk of cardiovascular events like heart attack and heart failure. In USA it is not banned but available with restricted use.

The animal studies had shown that Pioglitazone cause urinary bladder tumour in male rats in a two year study. Based on some studies US FDA in 2010 issued safety warning that there has been evidence to suggest that an increased risk of bladder cancer in patients with largest exposure of Pioglitazone and those taking highest cumulative dose. Further on 04 August 2011 warned the Healthcare Professionals and also a change in product label that the use of the drug for more than one year may be associated with increased risk of bladder cancer. It recommended "Not to use Pioglitazone in patients with active bladder cancer" and "Use with caution in patients with a prior history of bladder cancer". The FDA calculated the risk as the use of Pioglitazone was associated with 27.5 excess cases of bladder cancer per one lakh patients using the drug for one year compared to those who never use Pioglitazone.

Worst Pills, Best Pills, an independent drug information bulletin of USA termed the drug, Pioglitazone, as do not use category drug. It advised the patients not to use this antidiabetic drug as it is associated with several other side effects like liver damage, weight gain, anaemia and heart failure in addition to the risk of bladder cancer. The safer alternatives like glimepiride, glipizide, glyburide, tolazamide, tolbutamide and metformin.

France had suspended the use of Pioglitazone and Germany recommended that no new patients be given Pioglitazone. Though there has been perceived of a potential safety risk there is no established causal relationship between the use of Pioglitazone and bladder cancer.

Pioglitazone with respect to Bladder Cancer [Source: PvPI Newsletter, August 2013 Issue]	
Country	**Regulatory Status**
India	The drug should not be used as first line therapy of diabetes. The manufacturers should mention box warning in bold red letters.
France	Banned in July 2011
United States	Label Warning like 'not to use in patients with active bladder cancer'.
Japan	Label Warning like 'not to use in patients with active bladder cancer'.
Germany	Label warning like 'due to slight increase of risk bladder cancer the doctors should not prescribe in patients with bladder cancer (visible blood in the urine'.
There were reports of 54 ADRs for the drug in Indian database comprising of facial oedema, hypoglycaemia, aggravated hypoglycaemia, oedema, oedema in legs, giddiness, hypotension and drowsiness. There was only one case of bladder carcinoma in Indian database against the reports of 1241 cases globally as of June 2013.	

In India, the Government of India, Ministry of Health and Family Welfare (CDSCO)'s ban was misfired inviting protests from all over. Finally, the Government tracked back 'it is re-looking at the whole issue'. The decision to notification suspending the use of the drug was issued without following the standard protocol. The Ministry had not consulted the highest technical body, DTAB and was the unilateral whimsical decision of the country's top drug regulatory body, central drugs standard control organization.

Millions of diabetic patients are with pioglitazone, a cost effective medicine. The sudden banning of the medicine causes not only panic but also inconvenience to the patient as well to doctors. The medicine is not only regulates the blood glucose level but has additional advantages of regulating triglyceride level. It seems eight cases of bladder cancer in patients with pioglitazone were observed and the case reports were published in a journal as the letter to the editor. This report is not as peer reviewed scientific publication. While the millions of patients are under pioglitazone, it is not known the observations of 8 cases are out of how many?? This was one of the issues in the controversial ban.

On review of the decision, Drugs and Technical Advisory Board (DTAB), recommended the continuing use of pioglitazone but with a warning. DTAB is the highest advisory board of experts that recommends the government on technical matters relating to medicines. Similar to the US warning, now it is recommended to restrict the dose to 30 mg and screening of patients every six months for side effects.

In an interesting incidence, the Japanese Pharmaceutical Company, Takeda, agreed to pay up to $2.4 billion to settle US suits against its actos (pioglitazone). It was alleged that it hid the cancer risk of the drug. Though the company seems to have not agreed to the allegation but went for out of court settlement as strategy to 'reduce financial uncertainties'. [Source: News Reports of 28th April 2015 appeared in various media].

Bibliography

1. Hashmi A., Pioglitazone suspension and its aftermath: A wake up call for the Indian drug regulatory authorities, J Pharmacol Pharmacother, 2013.
2. Guru Prasad Mohanta, Much ado, nothing? Orissa Post, 09 August 2013.
3. GSR 379 (E), Ministry of Health and Family Welfare, 18 June 2013, The Gazette of India, New Delhi No. 294, June 18, 2013.
4. GSR 520 (E), Ministry of Health and Family Welfare, 31 July 2013, The Gazette of India, New Delhi No. 384, July 31, 2013.
5. Bladder Cancer Warning for Pioglitazone, Worst Pills Best Pills Newsletter, November 2011.
6. R. Prasad, Diabetes drug: 'May be I erred in my judgement', The Hindu, 17th July 2013.
7. Guru Prasad Mohanta, Pioglitazone: Unneeded Controversy, The Pharma Review, May – June 2014.

Chapter 14

Case Studies on Causality Assessment

"Tell me and I will forget, Show me and I will remember, Involve me and I will understand".

Confucius

CASE STUDY – 1 [Certain]

Mr. G, 42 year old, was admitted in surgery ward after haemorrhoidectomy. He was known allergic to Aspirin, Paracetamol and Diclofenac. Patient had no known comorbidity at the time of surgery.

His treating surgeon decided to put him on Inj Cefaperazone + Sulbactum 1.5 g q12h and Inj Metronidazole 0.5 g q12h; and Inj Ketorolac. Cefaperazone, Sulbactum and Metronidazole were meant for preventing post surgical infection and Ketorolac for the management of post operative pain. Prior to IV administration, test dose of Ketorolac was given intradermally to rule out allergic reactions, if any, and was put on observation for 30 minutes. Patient was found to be normal with no signs of allergic reaction. Following the test for allergic reaction, he was administered Ketorolac.

Following Inj Ketorolac 30 mg IV infusion, within 15 minutes patient started developing erythema on face which soon progressed to upper limbs and trunk followed by periorbital oedema, dyspnoea and hypotension (BP = 80/60 mmHg). The infusion was immediately stopped following which gradual symptomatic improvement was noticed.

Clinician made an impression about the reaction as acute anaphylaxis. Assess the causality for the given reaction using Naranjo's Probability Scale and explain.

S. No.	Questions	Yes	No	Don't know	Score
1	Are there previous *conclusive* reports on this reaction?	+1	0	0	+1
2	Did the adverse event appear after the suspected drug was administered?	+2	-1	0	+2
3	Did the adverse reaction improve when the drug was discontinued or a *specific* antagonist was administered?	+1	0	0	+1
4	Did the adverse event reappear when the drug was re-administered?	+2	-1	0	0
5	Are there alternative causes (other than the drug) that could on their own have caused the reaction?	-1	+2	0	+2
6	Did the reaction reappear when a placebo was given?	-1	+1	0	0
7	Was the drug detected in blood (or other fluids) in concentrations known to be toxic?	+1	0	0	0
8	Was the reaction more severe when the dose was increased or less severe when the dose was decreased?	+1	0	0	0
9	Did the patient have a similar reaction to the same or similar drugs in *any* previous exposure?	+1	0	0	+1
10	Was the adverse event confirmed by any objective evidence?	+1	0	0	+1
TOTAL SCORE					+8

This patient was known allergic to multiple drugs and had high risk in developing reaction with similar class of drugs as mentioned above. He had no other medically relevant co-morbidity. The reaction was clinically (objective) evident, had obvious and plausible time relationship with medication administered. IV infusion of ketorolac was stopped immediately after onset of reaction and the patient started recovering gradually within an hour after infusion was stopped.

Item no. 4 and 6 have been assigned 0 indicating don't know (note that don't know is to be used sparingly, here it denotes not applicable). Total score is +8 using Naranjo scale but Anaphylaxis falls in special category of causality where usual parameter like rechallenge is not applicable. In this case suspected drug was given in the form IV infusion and therefore dechallenge can be applied. Remember that Rechallenge is never done in serious reactions like this in the interest of patient safety (it is unethical too). Causality for anaphylaxis is always assessed as ***Certain.***

Using WHO scale for this example

(Consider the points written in **bold** *while working with WHO scale).*

Patient did not show any sign of reaction with test dose but with full dose. There is obvious and **reasonable time relationship** with drug intake and the reaction. It is **less likely** to be **attributed** to **disease** and the **other concomitant drug** as well. But ketorolac is highly suspected because patient has history of reaction for similar drugs and reaction (**anaphylaxis**) occurred within 15 minutes while on ketorolac. Only because patient was on IV infusion drug was stopped. Correlating all these data in the given case, the given example falls under the category ***"Certain" (special category).***

CASE STUDY – 2 [Certain]

A 31 year old fisherwoman weighing 49 kg, a known case of Pulmonary Tuberculosis, was with regimen CAT II ATT (oral Isoniazid 300 mg, Rifampicin 450 mg, Pyrazinamide 1500 mg, Ethambutol 1200 mg and inj Streptomycin 750 mg) since 15/01/15. She was neither receiving any concomitant drugs nor had any known co-morbidity. Family history of lymph node TB is known in her sister and brother. On 30/01/15 she came to dermatology OPD having developed generalized itching and rashes all over the body including face, numbness and swelling of lips. Patient was immediately admitted suspecting an ATT drugs induced ADR. She was symptomatically treated with Inj Avil and calamine lotion. On 4/02/15 she was symptomatically better and stable hence the physician decided to restart individual ATT drugs (same dose and brand was administered) considering her medical condition. It was found that the patient tolerated Isoniazid and Rifampicin but she developed generalized rash and itching all over the body within 2 hours following oral Pyrazinamide and dizziness, numbness, swelling of lips following inj Streptomycin. This time reaction was more severe than previous episode. Hence ***clinician made an impression that patient is allergic to Pyrazinamide and Streptomycin***. Offending drugs were stopped and patient was put on modified ATT drug regimen.

(*Note*: ATT means anti-tubercular treatment; CAT stands for Category)

Assess the causality for the given reaction using Naranjo's Probability Scale and explain.

S. No.	Questions	Yes	No	Don't know	Score
1	Are there previous *conclusive* reports on this reaction?	+1	0	0	+1
2	Did the adverse event appear after the suspected drug was administered?	+2	-1	0	+2
3	Did the adverse reaction improved when the drug was discontinued or a *specific* antagonist was administered?	+1	0	0	+1
4	Did the adverse event reappear when the drug was re-administered?	+2	-1	0	+2
5	Are there alternative causes (other than the drug) that could on their own have caused the reaction?	-1	+2	0	+2
6	Did the reaction reappear when a placebo was given?	-1	+1	0	0
7	Was the drug detected in blood (or other fluids) in concentrations known to be toxic?	+1	0	0	0
8	Was the reaction more severe when the dose was increased or less severe when the dose was decreased?	+1	0	0	+1
9	Did the patient have a similar reaction to the same or similar drugs in *any* previous exposure?	+1	0	0	0
10	Was the adverse event confirmed by any objective evidence?	+1	0	0	+1
	TOTAL SCORE				+10

The event was clinically specific and date of drug administration and onset of reaction had plausible time relationship. Patient was not on any concomitant drugs. Dechallenge is considered positive since patient recovered symptomatically in five days after withdrawal of the suspected drug. Rechallenge was done using one drug at a time to identify the culprit drug/s. It was found that following administration of Pyrazinamide as well as Streptomycin reactions reappeared and that they were more severe than the previous episode. Therefore, it was confirmed that the offending agents were Pyrazinamide and Streptomycin.

As the total score is +10, the causality is attributed as **Certain**.

[Always remember, "**Rechallenge**" means same drug, brand, dose and frequency. If not it is categorized as "reintroduction" and therefore assessment may change to ***Probable.***]

*Using **WHO** scale for this example*

*(Consider the points in **Bold** while working with WHO scale).*

In the above case, there is **plausible time relationship** with drug intake and reaction. There is **no correlation** with the disease and both **dechallenge** and **rechallenge** are positive for pyrazinamide and streptomycin; therefore, assessed as "***Certain***"

CASE STUDY – 3 [Probable]

A 65 year old female patient, a known case of COPD for last four years, was admitted in medicine wing of hospital with complaint of severe acute bronchospasm. Her weight was 58 kg. She was not known to have any drug allergy.

She was given the following medications after admission:

- Nebulizer Salbutamol 2.5 mg q6h
- Inj Aminophylline 300 mg dissolved in 20 ml of 5% dextrose over 20 minutes
- Inj Ampicillin 1g q6h
- Inj Furosemide 40 mg IV BD (last dose to be given by 4 pm)

At night 8 pm a duty physician observed disorientation and drowsiness in patient and he immediately ordered tests for serum electrolytes. The laboratory report showed a decreased levels of Sodium and Potassium: Serum Na^+ =114 mmol/L, Serum K^+=2.9 mmol/L. Physician suspected it to be **drug induced hyponatremia and hypokalemia due to Inj Furosemide;** thereby, the patient was given Inj. Potassium chloride. Additionally high salt in diet was also advised. (Note that the drug was not withdrawn considering furosemide as first line drug for peripheral oedema in COPD patients). After 7 days, serum electrolytes returned to normal levels (Serum Na^+=135 mmol/L, Serum K^+=3.8 mmol/L). Therefore, patient recovered.

Assess the causality for the given reaction using Naranjo's Probability Scale and explain.

S. No.	Questions	Yes	No	Don't know	Score
1	Are there previous *conclusive* reports on this reaction?	+1	0	0	+1
2	Did the adverse event appear after the suspected drug was administered?	+2	-1	0	+2
3	Did the adverse reaction improve when the drug was discontinued or a *specific* antagonist was administered?	+1	0	0	+1
4	Did the adverse event reappear when the drug was re-administered?	+2	-1	0	0
5	Are there alternative causes (other than the drug) that could on their own have caused the reaction?	-1	+2	0	+2
6	Did the reaction reappear when a placebo was given?	-1	+1	0	0
7	Was the drug detected in blood (or other fluids) in concentrations known to be toxic?	+1	0	0	0
8	Was the reaction more severe when the dose was increased or less severe when the dose was decreased?	+1	0	0	0
9	Did the patient have a similar reaction to the same or similar drugs in *any* previous exposure?	+1	0	0	0
10	Was the adverse event confirmed by any objective evidence?	+1	0	0	+1
	TOTAL SCORE				+7

Patient was on various concomitant drugs but the reaction was more specific to Furosemide due to its pharmacological action. Suspected drug was not withdrawn considering critical condition of patient but Dechallenge is considered positive as patient recovered symptomatically in 7 days after intervention (Inj. Potassium chloride and additional high salt in diet).

As Naranjo's algorithm score sums to +7, its causality category is "Probable".

*Using **WHO** scale for this example*

(Consider the points in bold while working with WHO scale).

It's found that there is **fluctuation in lab data** with a **reasonable time relationship** with drug intake. The reaction is **less likely** to be attributed to disease as well. Also in this case, drug was not withdrawn considering it as important in the patient treatment regimen, but the **reaction was treated** for which patient responded positively which also means that **dechallenge is positive**. Correlating all these data in the given case, the given example falls under the category ***"Probable".***

Case Study – 4 [Probable]

A 51 year old male patient has been recently diagnosed with Rheumatoid Arthritis. His clinician put him on oral sulfasalazine 500 mg, since 09/1/15. Along with that oral methyl prednisolone 4 mg was also added to the regimen. Fifteen days later (23/01/15) the patient was brought to the emergency ward having developed generalized exanthematous rash, maculopapular in nature, red raised lesions associated with intermittent episodes of fever. On examination, the patient was also found to have hepatomegaly. His laboratory tests showed elevated levels of ALP (346 IU/L) and AEC (380 cells/cumm). Immediately drug sulfasalazine was stopped and the reactions were treated symptomatically. The patient recovered on 31/1/15 and was discharged with Methotrexate replacing sulfasalazine. He was called again after 15 days for a review and found to be well tolerating the current regimen.

[ALP= Alkaline Phosphatase, AEC= Absolute Eosinophil Count]

Clinician made an impression as drug hypersensitivity syndrome due to sulfasalazine. Assess the causality for the given reaction using Naranjo's Probability Scale and explain.

S. No.	Questions	Yes	No	Don't know	Score
1	Are there previous *conclusive* reports on this reaction?	+1	0	0	+1
2	Did the adverse event appear after the suspected drug was administered?	+2	-1	0	+2
3	Did the adverse reaction improve when the drug was discontinued or a *specific* antagonist was administered?	+1	0	0	+1
4	Did the adverse event reappear when the drug was re-administered?	+2	-1	0	0
5	Are there alternative causes (other than the drug) that could on their own have caused the reaction?	-1	+2	0	+2

Contd...

S. No.	Questions	Yes	No	Don't know	Score
6	Did the reaction reappear when a placebo was given?	-1	+1	0	0
7	Was the drug detected in blood (or other fluids) in concentrations known to be toxic?	+1	0	0	0
8	Was the reaction more severe when the dose was increased or less severe when the dose was decreased?	+1	0	0	0
9	Did the patient have a similar reaction to the same or similar drugs in *any* previous exposure?	+1	0	0	0
10	Was the adverse event confirmed by any objective evidence?	+1	0	0	+1
TOTAL SCORE					+7

The above event was clinically specific; date of drug administration and onset of event was known; thus establishing plausible time relationship. Patient was on oral methyl prednisolone concomitantly but the reaction is most commonly known to occur due to sulfasalazine. Drug was immediately withdrawn on admission suspecting drug hypersensitivity syndrome and treated symptomatically. Patient recovered fully within a week and discharged with methotrexate. Dechallenge in this case is considered positive as patient recovered symptomatically in 7 days after intervention and was discharged with another effective drug .

As Naranjo's algorithm scores to **+7**, the causality falls under category "***Probable***".

*Using **WHO** scale for this example:*

*(Consider the points in **Bold** while working with WHO scale).*

Patient experienced **reaction** with sulfasalazine and lab data also fluctuated with reasonable **time relationship** of drug intake. The reaction **is less likely** to be attributed to disease and concomitant drug as well. In this case, the suspected drug was **withdrawn** and treated symptomatically following which patient **recovered**. The suspected drug was replaced with another effective drug and patient seemed to be normal. Hence, from the above points we can conclude that the case falls under the category *"**Probable**"*.

CASE STUDY – 5 [Possible]

A 16 year old ovarian cancer patient had completed 3 cycles of chemotherapy regimen consisting of Inj. Bleomycin, Etoposide and Cisplatin from a Private hospital. Third cycle of chemotherapy was completed on 16/03/15. Later, on 29/03/15 she was brought in Dept of Respiratory Medicine. At the time of admission, she had dyspnea on exertion (severity: grade III), orthopnea, cough with mucoid sputum and intermittent low grade fever.

On chest examination: Bilaterally fine crackle is heard.

Past history: No history of exposure to pets, wheezing, breathlessness and chest pain since childhood.

High resolution computed tomography of thorax suggested bilateral ground glass appearance consistent with Bleomycin toxicity.

Her treating physician diagnosed reaction as ***Bleomycin Induced Lung Fibrosis***. Condition of patient further deteriorated during her hospital stay and **expired** after fifteen days.

*Assess **causality for given case using Naranjo's probability scale and explain.***

S. No.	Questions	Yes	No	Don't know	Score
1	Are there previous *conclusive* reports on this reaction?	+1	0	0	+1
2	Did the adverse event appear after the suspected drug was administered?	+2	-1	0	+2
3	Did the adverse reaction improve when the drug was discontinued or a *specific* antagonist was administered?	+1	0	0	0
4	Did the adverse event reappear when the drug was re-administered?	+2	-1	0	0
5	Are there alternative causes (other than the drug) that could on their own have caused the reaction?	-1	+2	0	+2
6	Did the reaction reappear when a placebo was given?	-1	+1	0	0
7	Was the drug detected in blood (or other fluids) in concentrations known to be toxic?	+1	0	0	0

Contd...

S. No.	Questions	Yes	No	Don't know	Score
8	Was the reaction more severe when the dose was increased or less severe when the dose was decreased?	+1	0	0	0
9	Did the patient have a similar reaction to the same or similar drugs in *any* previous exposure?	+1	0	0	0
10	Was the adverse event confirmed by any objective evidence?	+1	0	0	+1
	TOTAL SCORE				+7

The **Naranjo scale** score sums to **+7** indicating that the reaction is **probable.** Though there is **plausible time relationship** with drug and reaction, there is no opportunity to see dechallenge as it is a death case. Death cases are always best coded as ***"Possible"*** if there is **plausible time relationship.** This applies with WHO scale also.

CASE STUDY – 6 [Possible]

A 40 year old male patient, with severe abdominal distension after having food, with complain of hiccups, was prescribed tablet Baclofen 5 mg on 02/2/15. After taking medication, he started vomiting. Patient was not on any other concomitant drug. He is chronic smoker and alcoholic since past 15 years and also a known case of TB. Drug was stopped on 05/2/15. Patient's recovered the next day. No other relevant medical conditions and lab details were mentioned at the time of reporting.

Physician diagnosed the condition as Drug induced ***Acute Gastric Enteritis.***

Assess causality for given case using Naranjo's probability scale and explain.

S. No.	Questions	Yes	No	Don't know	Score
1	Are there previous *conclusive* reports on this reaction?	+1	0	0	+1
2	Did the adverse event appear after the suspected drug was administered?	+2	-1	0	+2

Contd...

S. No.	Questions	Yes	No	Don't know	Score
3	Did the adverse reaction improve when the drug was discontinued or a *specific* antagonist was administered?	+1	0	0	+1
4	Did the adverse event reappear when the drug was re-administered?	+2	-1	0	0
5	Are there alternative causes (other than the drug) that could on their own have caused the reaction?	-1	+2	0	-1
6	Did the reaction reappear when a placebo was given?	-1	+1	0	0
7	Was the drug detected in blood (or other fluids) in concentrations known to be toxic?	+1	0	0	0
8	Was the reaction more severe when the dose was increased or less severe when the dose was decreased?	+1	0	0	0
9	Did the patient have a similar reaction to the same or similar drugs in *any* previous exposure?	+1	0	0	0
10	Was the adverse event confirmed by any objective evidence?	+1 [Vomiting in this case]	0	0	+1
	TOTAL SCORE				+4

Using Naranjo's probability scale the above reaction scored +4 which falls under the category "***Possible ADR***". There is no much detail available for this patient to assess. He is a chronic smoker and alcoholic; and therefore, vomiting is a common symptom of acute gastritis in such patients. Though the patient is a known case of TB, his medications are not known.

One cannot properly assess for any possible association of any drug with the reaction (various conditions are attributed to the cause).

The same explanation applies for ***WHO's assessment scale*** as well.

CASE STUDY – 7 [Un-assessable]

A 27 year old male patient went to a private physician nearby his locality with complaints of red eyes. The physician prescribed him an eye ointment diagnosing the condition as viral conjunctivitis. After a week the patient came to government hospital having developed fixed drug eruption. He also gave history of intake of medication for headache and ayurvedic drug for persisting knee pain. He had no prescription with him to identify the drugs when he came to hospital following the event.

Assess the causality for the given reaction using Naranjo's Probability Scale and explain.

S. No.	Questions	Yes	No	Don't know	Score
1	Are there previous *conclusive* reports on this reaction?	+1	0	0	0
2	Did the adverse event appear after the suspected drug was administered?	+2	-1	0	0
3	Did the adverse reaction improve when the drug was discontinued or a *specific* antagonist was administered?	+1	0	0	0
4	Did the adverse event reappear when the drug was re-administered?	+2	-1	0	0
5	Are there alternative causes (other than the drug) that could on their own have caused the reaction?	-1	+2	0	0
6	Did the reaction reappear when a placebo was given?	-1	+1	0	0
7	Was the drug detected in blood (or other fluids) in concentrations known to be toxic?	+1	0	0	0
8	Was the reaction more severe when the dose was increased or less severe when the dose was decreased?	+1	0	0	0
9	Did the patient have a similar reaction to the same or similar drugs in *any* previous exposure?	+1	0	0	0
10	Was the adverse event confirmed by any objective evidence?	+1	0	0	0
	TOTAL SCORE				0

Sufficient data on drugs used prior to the event is not available. The Patient has got no evidence (prescription) for verification of drugs taken. Hence score is "0" and the relationship is "***unassessable***".

[Contributed by Dr. J. Ponni, Pharm.D.]

Appendices

(a) ADR Reporting Form, National Pharmacovigilance Programme of India

SUSPECTED ADVERSE DRUG REACTION REPORTING FORM

For VOLUNTARY reporting of Adverse Drug Reactions by healthcare professionals

INDIAN PHARMACOPOEIA COMMISSION
(National Coordination Centre-Pharmacovigilance Programme of India)
Ministry of Health & Family Welfare
Government of India
Sector-23, Raj Nagar, Ghaziabad-201002
www.ipc.nic.in

(AMC/ NCC Use only)
AMC Report No.
Worldwide Unique

A. PATIENT INFORMATION

1. Patient Initials ______	2. Age at time of Event or date of birth ______	3. Sex ☐ M ☐ F 4. Weight ___Kgs

12. Relevant tests / laboratory data with dates

B. SUSPECTED ADVERSE REACTION

5. Date of reaction started (dd/mm/yyyy)

6. Date of recovery (dd/mm/yyyy)

7. Describe reaction or problem

13. Other relevant history including pre-existing medical conditions (e.g. allergies, race, pregnancy, smoking, alcohol use, hepatic/ renal dysfunction etc)

14. Seriousness of the reaction

- ☐ Death (dd/mm/yyyy)
- ☐ Life threatening
- ☐ Hospitalization/prolonged
- ☐ Disability
- ☐ Congenital-anomaly
- ☐ Required intervention to prevent permanent impairment / damage
- ☐ Other (specify)

15. Outcomes

- ☐ Fatal
- ☐ Continuing
- ☐ Recovering
- ☐ Recovered
- ☐ Unknown
- ☐ Other (specify)

C. SUSPECTED MEDICATION(S)

S.No	8. Name (brand and /or generic name)	Manufacturer (if known)	Batch No./ Lot No. (if known)	Exp. Date (if known))	Dose used	Route used	Frequency	Therapy dates (if known, give duration)		Reason for use of prescribed for
								Date started	Date stopped	
i.										
ii.										
iii.										
iv.										

S.No As per C	9. Reaction abated after drug stopped or dose reduced					10. Reaction reappeared after reintroduction				
	Yes	No	Unknown	NA	Reduced dose	Yes	No	Unknown	NA	If reintroduced dose
i.										
ii.										
iii.										
iv.										

11. Concomitant medical product including self medication and herbal remedies with therapy dates (exclude those used to treat reaction)

D. REPORTER (see confidentiality section on first page)

16. Name and Professional Address : ______________________

Pin code: ________E-mail ______________________

Tel. No. (with STD code): ______________________

Occupation ______________Signature ______________

17. Causality Assessment	18. Date of this report (dd/mm/yyyy)

ADVICE ABOUT REPORTING

- **Report adverse experiences with medications**
- **Report serious adverse reactions. A reaction is serious when the patient outcome is:**
  - death
  - life-threatening (real risk of dying)
  - hospitalization (initial or prolonged)
  - disability (significant, persistent or permanent
  - congenital anomaly
  - required intervention to prevent permanent impairment or damage
- **Report even if:**
  - You're not certain the product caused adverse reaction
  - You don't have all the details, however, point nos. **1, 5, 7, 8, 11, 15, 16 & 18** (see reverse) are essentially required.
- **Who can report:**
  - Any health care professional (Doctors including Dentists, Nurses and Pharmacists)
- **Where to report:**
  - Please return the completed form to the nearest **Adverse drug reaction Monitoring Centre** (AMC) or to **National Coordinating Centre**
  - A list of nationwide AMCs is available at: http://ipc.nic.in and also at http://cdsco.nic.in/pharmacovigilance.htm
- **What happens to the submitted information:**
  - Information provided in this form is handled in strict confidence. The causality assessment is carried out at Adverse Drug Reaction Monitoring Centres (AMCs) by using WHO-UMC scale. The analyzed forms are forwarded to the National Coordinating Centre through the ADR database. Finally the data is analyzed and forwarded to the Global Pharmacovigilance Database managed by WHO Uppsala Monitoring Center in Sweden.
  - The reports are periodically reviewed by the National Coordinating Centre (PvPI). The information generated on the basis of these reports helps in continuous assessment of the benefit-risk ratio of medicines.
  - The information is submitted to the Steering Committee of PvPI constituted by the Ministry of Health and Family Welfare. The Committee is entrusted with the responsibility to review the data and suggest any interventions that may be required.

Suspected Adverse Drug Reaction Reporting Form

For VOLUNTARY reporting of suspected adverse drug reactions by health care professionals

सत्यमेव जयते

IPC

National Coordinating Centre
Pharmacovigilance Programme of India
India Pharmacopoeia Commission
Ministry of Health & Family Welfare
Government of India
Sector-23, Raj Nagar, Ghaziabad-201002
Tel.:0120-2783400, 2783401, 2783392,
FAX: 0120-2783311
www.ipc.nic.in

Pharmacovigilance Programme of India for Assuring Drug Safety

Confidentiality: The patient's identity is held in strict confidence and protected to the fullest extent. Programme staff is not ex-pected to and will not disclose the reporter's identity in response to a request from the public. Submission of a report does not constitute an admission that medical personnel or manufacturer or the product caused or contributed to the reaction.

(b) ADR Reporting Form for Patient's use, National Pharmacovigilance Programme of India

MEDICINES SIDE EFFECT REPORTING FORM (FOR CONSUMERS)

Indian Pharmacopoeia Commission, National Coordination Centre- Pharmacovigilance Programme of India, Ministry of Health & Family Welfare, Government of India.

1.Patient Details

Patient Initials: ☐☐ | Gender (√): Male ☐ Female ☐ Other ☐ | Age (Year or Month) :

2. Health Information

a. Reason(s) for taking medicine(s)(Disease/Symptoms):

b. Medicines Advised by (√): Doctor ☐ Pharmacist ☐ Friends/Relatives ☐ Self (Past disease experienced/No past disease experienced) ☐

3. Details of Person Reporting the Side Effect

Name (Optional):

Address:

Telephone No: | Email:

4. Details of Medicine Taking/Taken

Name of Medicines	Quantity of Medicines taken (e.g. 250 mg, Two times a day)	Expiry Date of Medicines	Date of Start of Medicines	Date of Stop of Medicines
			dd/mm/yy	dd/mm/yy
			dd/mm/yy	dd/mm/yy
			dd/mm/yy	dd/mm/yy

Dosage form (√) : Tablet ☐ Capsule ☐ Injection ☐ Oral Liquids ☐ If Others (Please Specify..................................)

5. About the Side Effect

When did the side effect start? dd/mm/yy | Side Effect is still Continuing (Yes/No): ☐

When did the side effect stop? dd/mm/yy

6.How bad was the Side Effect? (Please √ the boxes that Apply)

☐ Did not affect daily activities | ☐ Affect daily activities

☐ Admitted to hospital | ☐ Death

☐ Others

7.Describe the Side Effect (What did you do to manage the side effect?)

This reporting is voluntary, has no legal implication and aims to improve patient safety. Your active participation is valuable. The information provided in this form will be forwarded to ADR Monitoring Centre for follow-up. You are requested to cooperate with the programme officials when they contact you for more details. Please do report even if you do not have all the information.

Please turn the page to read the instructions

Send your report by mail or Fax to	
Pharmacovigilance Programme of India National Coordination Centre, Indian Pharmacopoeia Commission, Ministry of Health & Family Welfare, Govt. of India Sector-23,Rajnagar,Ghaziabad-201002.Uttar Pradesh Tel.:0120-2783400, 2783401, 2783392 FAX: 0120-2783311 Email: pvpi.compat@gmail.com For more information visit us at *www.ipc.gov.in*	**Call us on Helpline** **1800180-3024** **(Toll Free)** **(9:00 AM to 5:30 PM, weekdays)**

Confidentiality: The patient's identity is held in strict confidence and protected to the fullest extent. Programme staff is not expected to and will not disclose the reporter's identity in response to a request from the public.

Instructions to Complete the Reporting Form

Section 1 - Patient Details

- ✓ In patient Initial, write first letter of the name and first letter of the surname (e.g. Pradeep Sharma-PS).
- ✓ Provide personal information (Gender, Age).

Section -2 Health Information

- ✓ Provide reason(s) for taking medicines and medicines advised by (Doctor, Pharmacists, Friends/ Relatives and Self).

Section 3 - Details of Person Reporting the Side Effect

- ✓ Provide the name (optional), address; telephone no. and email are necessary to assess the report.

Section 4 - Details of the Medicines Taking/Taken

- ✓ Give all details about the Medicines (Name of Medicines, Quantity of Medicines taken, Expiry Date, start and stop date of Medicines) that have caused side effect.
- ✓ Please provide Dosage form (Tablets, Capsule, injections, Oral liquid) and if others please specify.

Section 5 - About the Side Effect

- ✓ Provide side effect start and stop dates and also specify whether the side effect is still continuing.

Section 6 - How bad was the Side Effect

- ✓ Please tick marks the appropriate boxes that apply.

Section 7- Describe the Side Effect

- ✓ Please describe the details of side effect and what treatment was taken to manage the side effect.

Thank you for taking the time to complete this form

(c) Guidance for Filling up the ADR Form

A. Patient Information

1. ***Patient initials:*** A reporter should only mention the initials of a patient instead of the full name. For e.g.: Madhu Gupta should be written as MG.
2. ***Age at time of event or date of birth:*** A reporter must report either the date of birth or age of the patient at the time the event or reaction occurred.
3. ***Sex:*** A reporter must mention the gender of the patient.
4. ***Weight:*** The weight of the patient should be in kilograms.

B. Suspected Adverse Reaction

5. ***Date of reaction started:*** A reporter must report the date on which the reaction was first observed.
6. ***Date of recovery:*** If the reaction recovered, the date on which the reaction recovered should be reported.
7. ***Describe reaction:*** A reporter must briefly describe the event in terms of nature, localization etc. For example patient developed erythematous maculopapular rash over upper and lower limbs.

C. Suspected Medications

8. The details of suspected medication(s) such as the *drug name (brand or generic name), manufacturer, batch no/lot no, expiry date, dose used, route used, frequency, dates of therapy started and stopped, and indication of use* must be provided by the reporter.
9. ***De-challenge details:*** A reporter must report the status of de-challenge as:
   - **'Yes'** - if reaction abated or reduced after de-challenge
   - **'No'** - if reaction did not abated after de-challenge
   - **'Unknown'** - if information on de-challenge is not confirmed or not known
   - **'Not Applicable' or 'NA'** - if de-challenge is not possible as in case of anaphylaxis, life threatening events, anaesthetic drugs or where a single dose is given.

- **'Reduced dose'** - If dose at which the reaction occurred is reduced

Note: Also mention the reduced dose

10. ***Re-challenge details:*** A reporter must report the status of re-challenge as:
    - **'Yes'** - if reaction reappeared after re-challenge
    - **'No'** - if reaction did not reappear after re-challenge
    - **'Unknown'** - if information on re-challenge is not confirmed or not known
    - **'Not Applicable' or 'NA'** - if re-challenge is not applicable as in the case of injections.
    - **'Re-introduced dose'**- If the drug is reintroduced is it a reduced dose or is it the same dose at which adverse event occurred initially.
11. ***Concomitant drugs:*** A reporter should include all the details of concomitant drugs including self medication, OTC medication, herbal remedies with therapy dates (start and stop date.)
12. ***Relevant tests/ laboratory data:*** A reporter must mention any laboratory data (if available) relevant to the adverse event that occurred.
13. ***Other relevant history:*** A reporter must mention any relevant history pertaining to the patient including pre-existing medical conditions (e.g. allergies, pregnancy, smoking, alcohol use, hepatic/renal dysfunction).
14. ***Seriousness of the reaction:*** If any event is serious in nature, a reporter must select the appropriate reason for seriousness:
    - **'Death'** - if the patient died due to the adverse event
    - **'Life-threatening'** - if patient was at substantial risk of dying because of the adverse event
    - **'Hospitalisation/prolonged'** - if the adverse event led to hospitalization or increased the hospital stay of the patient
    - **'Disability'** - if the adverse event resulted in a substantial disruption of a person's ability to conduct normal life functions

- **'Congenital anomaly'** - if exposure of drug prior to conception or during pregnancy may have resulted in an adverse outcome in the child.
- **'Required intervention to prevent permanent impairment/damage'** - if medical or surgical intervention was necessary to preclude permanent impairment of a body function, or prevent permanent damage to a body structure
- **'Other'** - when the event does not fit the other outcomes, but the event may put the patient at risk and may require medical or surgical intervention to prevent one of the other outcomes. Examples include serious blood dyscrasias (blood disorders) or seizures/convulsions that do not result in hospitalization, development of drug dependence or drug abuse

15. ***Outcomes:*** The reporter must tick the outcome of the event as:
    - **'Fatal'** - if the patient dies due to the adverse event
    - **'Continuing'** - if the patient is continuing to have the symptoms of the adverse event which occurred
    - **'Recovering'** - if the patient is recovering from the existing adverse event
    - **'Recovered'** - if the patient has recovered from the event
    - **'Unknown'** - if the outcome is not known

D. Reporter

16. ***Name and Professional address:*** A reporter must mention his/her name and professional address on the form. The identity of the reporter will be maintained confidential
17. ***Causality assessment:*** The reporter (if trained) must perform the causality assessment.
18. ***Date of report:*** Mention the date on which he/she reported the adverse event.

***Note*:** For quality reporting of ICSRs all the above mentioned fields are essential. In case of incomplete information, the reporter must take care that at least mandatory fields are present. Following are the mandatory fields for a valid case report:

- ***Patient information:*** initials, age at onset of reaction, gender.
- ***Suspected adverse reaction:*** A reaction term(s), date of onset of reaction.
- ***Suspected medication:*** Drug(s) name, dose, date of therapy started, indication of use, seriousness, outcome, de-challenge and re-challenge details.
- ***Reporter:*** Name and address, causality assessment, date of report.

(d) ADR Reporting Form, CIOMS

CIOMS FORM

SUSPECT ADVERSE REACTION REPORT

I. REACTION INFORMATION

1. PATIENT INITIALS (first, last)	1a. COUNTRY	2. DATE OF BIRTH			2a. AGE	3. SEX	4-6 REACTION ONSET			8-12 CHECK ALL APPROPRIATE TO ADVERSE REACTION
		Day	Month	Year	Years		Day	Month	Year	
7 + 13 DESCRIBE REACTION(S) (including relevant tests/lab data)										☐ PATIENT DIED ☐ INVOLVED OR PROLONGED INPATIENT HOSPITALISATION ☐ INVOLVED PERSISTENCE OR SIGNIFICANT DISABILITY OR INCAPACITY ☐ LIFE THREATENING

II. SUSPECT DRUG(S) INFORMATION

14. SUSPECT DRUG(S) (include generic name)		20 DID REACTION ABATE AFTER STOPPING DRUG? ☐ YES ☐ NO ☐ NA
15. DAILY DOSE(S)	16. ROUTE(S) OF ADMINISTRATION	21. DID REACTION REAPPEAR AFTER REINTRODUCTION? ☐ YES ☐ NO ☐ NA
17. INDICATION(S) FOR USE		
18. THERAPY DATES (from/to)	19. THERAPY DURATION	

III. CONCOMITANT DRUG(S) AND HISTORY

22. CONCOMITANT DRUG(S) AND DATES OF ADMINISTRATION (exclude those used to treat reaction)
23. OTHER RELEVANT HISTORY (e.g. diagnostics, allergics, pregnancy with last month of period, etc.)

IV. MANUFACTURER INFORMATION

24a. NAME AND ADDRESS OF MANUFACTURER		
	24b. MFR CONTROL NO.	
24c. DATE RECEIVED BY MANUFACTURER	24d. REPORT SOURCE ☐ STUDY ☐ LITERATURE ☐ HEALTH PROFESSIONAL	
DATE OF THIS REPORT	25a. REPORT TYPE ☐ INITIAL ☐ FOLLOWUP	

(e) ADR Reporting Form, Yellow Card, UK

In Confidence

YellowCard
COMMISSION ON HUMAN MEDICINES (CHM)

It's easy to report online at
www.mhra.gov.uk/yellowcard

MHRA

REPORT OF SUSPECTED ADVERSE DRUG REACTIONS

If you suspect an adverse reaction may be related to one or more drugs/vaccines/complementary remedies, please complete this Yellow Card. See 'Adverse reactions to drugs' section in the British National Formulary (BNF) or **www.mhra.gov.uk/yellowcard** for guidance. Do not be put off reporting because some details are not known.

PATIENT DETAILS Patient Initials:__________ Sex: M / F Is the patient pregnant? Y / N Ethnicity:______________

Age (at time of reaction):_______ Weight (kg):________ Identification number (e.g. Practice or Hospital Ref):______________

SUSPECTED DRUG(S)/VACCINE(S)

Drug/Vaccine (Brand if known)	Batch	Route	Dosage	Date started	Date stopped	Prescribed for

SUSPECTED REACTION(S) Please describe the reaction(s) and any treatment given. (Please attach additional pages if necessary):

Outcome
- Recovered ☐
- Recovering ☐
- Continuing ☐
- Other ☐

Date reaction(s) started:______________ Date reaction(s) stopped: ______________

Do you consider the reactions to be serious? Yes / No

If yes, please indicate why the reaction is considered to be serious (please tick all that apply):

- ☐ Patient died due to reaction
- ☐ Involved or prolonged inpatient hospitalisation
- ☐ Life threatening
- ☐ Involved persistent or significant disability or incapacity
- ☐ Congenital abnormality
- Medically significant; please give details: ______________

If the reactions were not serious according to the categories above, how bad was the suspected reaction?

☐ Mild ☐ Unpleasant, but did not affect everyday activities ☐ Bad enough to affect everyday activities

OTHER DRUG(S) (including self-medication and complementary remedies)

Did the patient take any other medicines/vaccines/complementary remedies in the last 3 months prior to the reaction? Yes / No

If yes, please give the following information if known:

Drug/Vaccine (Brand if known)	Batch	Route	Dosage	Date started	Date stopped	Prescribed for

Additional relevant information e.g. medical history, test results, known allergies, rechallenge (if performed). For reactions relating to use of a medicine during pregnancy please state all other drugs taken during pregnancy, the last menstrual period, information on previous pregnancies, ultrasound scans, any delivery complications, birth defects or developmental concerns.

Please list any medicines obtained from the internet:

REPORTER DETAILS

Name and Professional Address:______________

Postcode:__________ Tel No:__________

Email:______________

Speciality:______________

Signature:__________ Date:__________

CLINICIAN (if not the reporter)

Name and Professional Address:______________

Postcode:__________ Tel No:__________

Email:______________

Speciality:______________

Date:______________

Information on adverse drug reactions received by the MHRA can be downloaded at **www.mhra.gov.uk/daps**
Stay up-to-date on the latest advice for the safe use of medicines with our monthly bulletin *Drug Safety Update* at **www.mhra.gov.uk/drugsafetyupdate**

Please attach additional pages if necessary. Send to: FREEPOST YELLOW CARD (no other address details required)

FREEPOST YELLOW CARD

SECOND FOLD HERE

GUIDELINES FOR YELLOW CARD REPORTING

Please use the Yellow Card Scheme to tell us about:

- **All** suspected adverse drug reactions **for new medicines** - identified by the black triangle ▼ symbol
- **All** suspected adverse drug reactions occurring **in children**, even if a medicine has been used off-label
- **All serious*** suspected adverse drug reactions for established vaccines and medicines, including unlicensed medicines, herbal remedies, and medicines used off-label
- **All medication errors** that **result in an adverse reaction**

*Reactions which are fatal, life-threatening, a congenital abnormality, disabling or incapacitating, result in or prolong hospitalisation, or medically significant are considered serious.

If you are unsure, please report anyway

For more information:

- Contact the Yellow Card Information Service on Freephone 0800 731 6789
- Visit the Yellow Card website – **www.mhra.gov.uk/yellowcard**

FIRST FOLD HERE

(f) ADR Reporting Form, MedWatch

Reset Form

U.S. Department of Health and Human Services

MEDWATCH

The FDA Safety Information and Adverse Event Reporting Program

For VOLUNTARY reporting of adverse events, product problems and product use errors

Page 1 of 3

Form Approved: OMB No. 0910-0291, Expires: 6/30/2015
See PRA statement on reverse.

FDA USE ONLY
Triage unit sequence #

PLEASE TYPE OR USE BLACK INK

A. PATIENT INFORMATION

1. Patient Identifier — In confidence
2. Age at Time of Event or Date of Birth:
3. Sex — ☐ Female ☐ Male
4. Weight — ____ lb or ____ kg

B. ADVERSE EVENT, PRODUCT PROBLEM OR ERROR

Check all that apply:

1. ☐ Adverse Event ☐ Product Problem (*e.g., defects/malfunctions*)
☐ Product Use Error ☐ Problem with Different Manufacturer of Same Medicine

2. Outcomes Attributed to Adverse Event (*Check all that apply*)
☐ Death: ________ (*mm/dd/yyyy*)
☐ Disability or Permanent Damage
☐ Life-threatening
☐ Congenital Anomaly/Birth Defect
☐ Hospitalization - initial or prolonged
☐ Other Serious (Important Medical Events)
☐ Required Intervention to Prevent Permanent Impairment/Damage (Devices)

3. Date of Event (*mm/dd/yyyy*)
4. Date of this Report (*mm/dd/yyyy*)

5. Describe Event, Problem or Product Use Error

(Continue on page 3)

6. Relevant Tests/Laboratory Data, Including Dates

(Continue on page 3)

7. Other Relevant History, Including Preexisting Medical Conditions (*e.g., allergies, race, pregnancy, smoking and alcohol use, liver/kidney problems, etc.*)

(Continue on page 3)

C. PRODUCT AVAILABILITY

Product Available for Evaluation? (*Do not send product to FDA*)
☐ Yes ☐ No ☐ Returned to Manufacturer on: ________ (*mm/dd/yyyy*)

D. SUSPECT PRODUCT(S)

1. Name, Strength, Manufacturer (*from product label*)
#1 Name:
Strength:
Manufacturer:
#2 Name:
Strength:
Manufacturer:

2. Dose or Amount — Frequency — Route
#1
#2

3. Dates of Use (*If unknown, give duration*) from/to (*or best estimate*)
#1
#2

4. Diagnosis or Reason for Use (*Indication*)
#1
#2

5. Event Abated After Use Stopped or Dose Reduced?
#1 ☐ Yes ☐ No ☐ Doesn't Apply
#2 ☐ Yes ☐ No ☐ Doesn't Apply

6. Lot #
#1
#2

7. Expiration Date
#1
#2

8. Event Reappeared After Reintroduction?
#1 ☐ Yes ☐ No ☐ Doesn't Apply
#2 ☐ Yes ☐ No ☐ Doesn't Apply

9. NDC # or Unique ID

E. SUSPECT MEDICAL DEVICE

1. Brand Name
2. Common Device Name
2b. Procode
3. Manufacturer Name, City and State
4. Model # — Lot #
Catalog # — Expiration Date (*mm/dd/yyyy*)
Serial # — Unique Identifier (UDI) #
5. Operator of Device
☐ Health Professional
☐ Lay User/Patient
☐ Other:
6. If Implanted, Give Date (*mm/dd/yyyy*)
7. If Explanted, Give Date (*mm/dd/yyyy*)
8. Is this a Single-use Device that was Reprocessed and Reused on a Patient?
☐ Yes ☐ No
9. If Yes to Item No. 8, Enter Name and Address of Reprocessor

F. OTHER (CONCOMITANT) MEDICAL PRODUCTS

Product names and therapy dates (exclude treatment of event)

(Continue on page 3)

G. REPORTER (*See confidentiality section on back*)

1. Name and Address
Name:
Address:
City: State: ZIP:
Phone # — E-mail
2. Health Professional? ☐ Yes ☐ No
3. Occupation
4. Also Reported to:
☐ Manufacturer
☐ User Facility
☐ Distributor/Importer
5. If you do NOT want your identity disclosed to the manufacturer, place an "X" in this box: ☐

FORM FDA 3500 (2/13) Submission of a report does not constitute an admission that medical personnel or the product caused or contributed to the event.

Delete Page

ADVICE ABOUT VOLUNTARY REPORTING

Detailed instructions available at: http://www.fda.gov/medwatch/report/consumer/instruct.htm

Report adverse events, product problems or product use errors with:

- Medications *(drugs or biologics)*
- Medical devices *(including in-vitro diagnostics)*
- Combination products *(medication & medical devices)*
- Human cells, tissues, and cellular and tissue-based products
- Special nutritional products *(dietary supplements, medical foods, infant formulas)*
- Cosmetics
- Food *(including beverages and ingredients added to foods)*

Report product problems - quality, performance or safety concerns such as:

- Suspected counterfeit product
- Suspected contamination
- Questionable stability
- Defective components
- Poor packaging or labeling
- Therapeutic failures (product didn't work)

-Fold Here-

Report SERIOUS adverse events. An event is serious when the patient outcome is:

- Death
- Life-threatening
- Hospitalization - initial or prolonged
- Disability or permanent damage
- Congenital anomaly/birth defect
- Required intervention to prevent permanent impairment or damage (devices)
- Other serious (important medical events)

Report even if:

- You're not certain the product caused the event
- You don't have all the details

How to report:

- Just fill in the sections that apply to your report
- Use section D for all products except medical devices
- Attach additional pages if needed
- Use a separate form for each patient
- Report either to FDA or the manufacturer *(or both)*

Other methods of reporting:

- 1-800-FDA-0178 - To FAX report
- 1-800-FDA-1088 - To report by phone
- www.fda.gov/medwatch/report.htm - To report online

If your report involves a serious adverse event with a device and it occurred in a facility outside a doctor's office, that facility may be legally required to report to FDA and/or the manufacturer. Please notify the person in that facility who would handle such reporting.

-Fold Here-

If your report involves a serious adverse event with a vaccine, call 1-800-822-7967 to report.

Confidentiality: The patient's identity is held in strict confidence by FDA and protected to the fullest extent of the law. FDA will not disclose the reporter's identity in response to a request from the public, pursuant to the Freedom of Information Act. The reporter's identity, including the identity of a self-reporter, may be shared with the manufacturer unless requested otherwise.

The information in this box applies only to requirements of the Paperwork Reduction Act of 1995

The burden time for this collection of information has been estimated to average 36 minutes per response, including the time to review instructions, search existing data sources, gather and maintain the data needed, and complete and review the collection of information. Send comments regarding this burden estimate or any other aspect of this collection of information, including suggestions for reducing this burden to:

Department of Health and Human Services
Food and Drug Administration
Office of Chief Information Officer
Paperwork Reduction Act (PRA) Staff
PRAStaff@fda.hhs.gov

Please DO NOT RETURN this form to the PRA Staff e-mail to the left.

OMB statement: "An agency may not conduct or sponsor, and a person is not required to respond to, a collection of information unless it displays a currently valid OMB control number."

U.S. DEPARTMENT OF HEALTH AND HUMAN SERVICES
Food and Drug Administration

FORM FDA 3500 (2/13) (Back) **Please Use Address Provided Below -- Fold in Thirds, Tape and Mail**

DEPARTMENT OF
HEALTH & HUMAN SERVICES

Public Health Service
Food and Drug Administration
Rockville, MD 20857

Official Business
Penalty for Private Use $300

NO POSTAGE NECESSARY IF MAILED IN THE UNITED STATES OR APO/FPO

BUSINESS REPLY MAIL

FIRST CLASS MAIL PERMIT NO. 946 ROCKVILLE MD

POSTAGE WILL BE PAID BY FOOD AND DRUG ADMINISTRATION

MEDWATCH
The FDA Safety Information and Adverse Event Reporting Program
Food and Drug Administration
5600 Fishers Lane
Rockville, MD 20852-9787

Reset Form | Delete Page

U.S. Department of Health and Human Services

MEDWATCH

The FDA Safety Information and Adverse Event Reporting Program

(CONTINUATION PAGE)

For VOLUNTARY reporting of adverse events and product problems

Page 3 of 3

B.5. **Describe Event or Problem** *(continued)*

Back to Form

B.6. **Relevant Tests/Laboratory Data, Including Dates** *(continued)*

Back to Form

B.7. **Other Relevant History, Including Preexisting Medical Conditions** *(e.g., allergies, race, pregnancy, smoking and alcohol use, hepatic/renal dysfunction, etc.) (continued)*

Back to Form

F. Concomitant Medical Products and Therapy Dates *(Exclude treatment of event) (continued)*

Back to Form

(g) ADR Reporting Form, Blue Card, Australia

Australian Government
Department of Health
Therapeutic Goods Administration

TGA use only

Report of suspected adverse reaction to medicines or vaccines

See statement about the collection and use of personal information overleaf, and please attach any additional data to this form

Patient initials or medical record number:	Sex: M ☐ F ☐ Weight (kg):	Date of birth or age:

Suspected medicine(s)/vaccine(s)

Medicine/vaccine (please use trade names; include batch number and AUST R or AUST L number if known)	**Dosage** (Dose number for vaccines eg 1st DTP)	Date begun	Date stopped	Reason for use

Other medicine(s)/vaccine(s) taken at the time of the reaction

Medicine/vaccine	**Dosage**	Date begun	Date stopped	Reason for use

Reaction(s): Date of onset of reaction (for vaccines time after administration): / /

Describe: (please provide as much detail as possible and include any results of relevant laboratory data and other investigations)

Seriousness: Life threatening ☐ Hospitalised ☐ Required a visit to doctor ☐

Treatment of reaction:

Outcome: Recovered ☐ ▶ Date: / / | Not yet recovered ☐ | Fatal ☐ ▶ Date: / / | Unknown ☐

Sequelae? No ☐ Yes ☐ ▶ Describe:

Reporting: Doctor ☐ Pharmacist ☐ Other ☐ | Contact details (email or phone)

Name:

Address:

Postcode: | Signature: | Date: / /

Thank you for taking the time to complete this form PTO

Report of suspected reaction to medicines or vaccines ("Blue card")

Privacy statement

Personal information:

Personal information in this report about a patient is collected and used for the purpose of assessing the safety of medicines under the *Therapeutic Goods Act 1989* (the Act). All reports are assessed and entered into the TGA's Australian Adverse Drugs Reactions System (the ADRS). That information in this report is only disclosed: (i) under subsection 61(3) of the Act to State and Territory Health Departments (if the information relates to vaccine events); or (ii) where the disclosure is otherwise required by, or authorised under, a law. For example, the Secretary of the Department of Health can release information from this report under subsection 61(7) of the Act if it is necessary to do so to ensure the safe use of the medicine, including to the company responsible for its supply in Australia.

The reporter's details are recorded in the ADRS so that they can be contacted if further information is required about the reported adverse event. Personal information about a reporter is only disclosed: (i) under subsection 61(3) of the Act to State and Territory Health Departments (if the information relates to vaccine events); or (ii) where the disclosure is otherwise required by, or authorised under, a law.

Adverse event information:

Specified kinds of information about reported adverse events can be released to the public by the Secretary under subsection 61(5C) of the Act. The information includes such details as the medicine reported to have been involved in an adverse event, and statistics such as the number of cases of reported adverse events relating to a medicine for any particular period of time. This information does not include any "personal information" within the meaning of the *Privacy Act 1988* - that is, information from which an individual's identity might be apparent or reasonably ascertainable.

Further information about how the TGA uses adverse event information that is reported to it is available at <www.tga.gov.au/reporting-problems>.

Fold here first (Please do not use staples on this form)

Phone: 1800 044 114 www.tga.gov.au/reporting-problems Email: adr.reports@tga.gov.au Fax: 02 6232 8392

What to report

You do not need to be certain, just suspicious!

Any information related to the reporter and patient identifiers is kept strictly confidential.

Adverse drug reaction reports should be submitted for prescription medicines, vaccines, over-the-counter medicines (medicines purchased without a prescription), and complementary medicines (herbal medicines, naturopathic and/or homoeopathic medicines, and nutritional supplements such as vitamins and minerals).

Please include timing of reactions relative to medicine administration where relevant.

The TGA particularly requests reports of:

- All suspected reactions to new medicines and vaccines
- All suspected drug interactions
- Unexpected reactions, that is not consistent with product information or labelling
- Serious reactions which are suspected of significantly affecting a patient's management, including reactions suspected of causing death, danger to life, admission to hospital, prolongation of hospitalisation, absence from productive activity, increased investigational or treatment costs, and birth defects.

Fold here second D1073 February 2015

Delivery Address:
PO Box 100
WODEN ACT 2606

No stamp required if posted in Australia

Medicines Safety Monitoring
Post-market Surveillance Branch
Reply Paid 100
WODEN ACT 2606

Glossary

Absolute Risk: Risk in a population of exposed persons. Absolute risk can be measured in over time or at a given time.

Adverse (Drug) Event: Any untoward medical occurrence that may present during treatment with a pharmaceutical product which does not necessarily have a causal relationship with the treatment. [An event is any new clinical experience that occurs after commencing treatment with a medicine regardless of its severity or seriousness and without judgement on its causality. Favourable events may be recorded as an indication of an unexpected therapeutic effect. ADR in a patient is an adverse outcome that is attributed to a suspected action of a drug while the Adverse Event is an adverse outcome that occurs after the use of a drug, *but which may or may not be linked to use of the drug*. All ADRs are Adverse (Drug) Events but the reverse is not true. All Adverse (Drug) Events are not necessarily ADRs]. Example of adverse drug event: Heart arrhythmia from discontinuing atenolol (whether or not is an error); Example of adverse drug reaction: skin rashes from nevirapine.

Adverse Drug Reaction (ADR): A response to a medicine that is noxious and unintended and occurs at doses normally used in man for prophylaxis, diagnosis, or therapy of disease, or for the modification of physiological function. The WHO definition excludes well known side effects. Side effects are usually noxious, unintended but expected in usual dose. But the ADR is not expected. This ADR definition does not include intentional or accidental poisoning or drug abuse too. [Adverse Drug Reaction and Adverse Drug Event are often used interchangeably. Adverse reaction refers to the patient point of view while adverse effect applies to the drug]. An adverse reaction, contrary to the adverse event, is characterised by the suspicion of a causal relationship between the drug and occurrence: judged possibly by reporting or reviewing by health professional. An ADR is always an ADE but ADE need not be ADR. ADE may be due to overdose caused by dispensing error.

Adverse Events Following Immunization (AEFI): Medical Incident that takes place after an immunization causes concern and is believed to have caused by immunization.

Attributable Risk: Difference between the risk in an exposed population (absolute risk) and the risk in an unexposed population. This is also known as excess risk.

Audit Finding(s): Results of the evaluation of the collected evidence against prefixed criteria.

Audit Plan: Description of activities and arrangement for an assessment.

Audit Programme: Set of one or more audits planned for a specific timeframe and for a specific purpose.

Audit Recommendation: Activities that the management might consider to rectify conditions that have gone away and to mitigate weaknesses in systems of management control. Audit recommendations should be positive and as specific as possible. They should also identify who is to act on them.

Audit: A systematic, disciplined, independent and documented process for obtaining evidence and evaluating it objectively to determine the extent of compliance to policies, procedures and requirements.

Benefit –Risk Analysis: Examination of the favourable and unfavourable results for undertaking a specific course of action.

Benefit: An estimated gain for an individual or population.

Bioethics: Ethical principles of biomedical research in human beings.

Causality Assessment: The evaluation of likelihood that a medicine was the causative agent of an observed adverse event.

Clinical Trial: Human experimentations for assessing the safety and efficacy of a medicinal product.

Cohort Event Monitoring: A prospective observational study of adverse events associated with one or more medicines.

Dechallenge: The withdrawal of the drug following suspected adverse drug reaction.

Effectiveness: The ability of the medicine to produce the desired beneficial effect in actual use.

Efficacy: The ability of the drug to produce the intended effects under ideal conditions of use.

Electronic Health Record Mining: Scanning of electronic health record for detecting desired information.

Individual Case Safety Report: A suspected adverse drug reaction report that occurred in an individual patient.

Informed Consent: Providing acceptance for participating in the research with full knowledge and understanding the risk and benefit.

Naranjo Probability Scale: A tool used to establish a relationship between an adverse event and the suspected drug.

Periodic Adverse Drug Experience Report [PADER]/Periodic Adverse Experience Report (PAER): Periodically developed safety data for submission to US FDA. These are previous format for submitting PSUR, now replaced with PBRER.

Periodic Benefit Risk Evaluation Report (PBRER): US FDA requirement to submit safety and benefit report at predetermined interval for a marketed product. This is a new format for submitting PSUR (now the term is changed).

Periodic Safety Update Report [PSUR]: A document periodically developed containing comprehensive worldwide safety data of a marketed product.

Pharmacogenetics: The use of genetic markers to maximise the safety and/or efficacy of drugs.

Pharmacovigilance: The science and activities relating to the detection, assessment, understanding and prevention of adverse effects or any other drug related problem.

Polypharmacy: The concomitant use of more than one drug.

Quality Adherence: Carrying out tasks and responsibilities in accordance with quality requirements.

Quality Assurance: The planned and systematic activities designed and carried out in a system so that the quality requirement for a programme or system is ensured.

Quality Control: Part of quality management focussed on fulfilling quality requirements like characteristics of a product, process or system.

Quality Improvements: Correcting and improving the structures and processes where necessary. This applies for the purpose of fulfilling quality requirements.

Quality of a Pharmacovigilance System: All characteristics of the pharmacovigilance system which are considered to be in consistent to the objectives of pharmacovigilance.

Quality Planning: Establishing structures and planning of integrated and consistent processes to fulfil quality requirements.

Quality Requirements: Those characteristics of a system likely to produce the desired outcome.

Quality System of a Pharmacovigilance System: The organisational structure, responsibilities, procedures and resources of the pharmacovigilance system responsible for quality outcomes.

Rechallenge: The drug is given again to the patient after withdrawal (following suspected adverse drug reaction) on complete recovery of ADR symptoms.

Record Linkage: Methods of assembling information contained in two or more records.

Relative Risk: The ratio of the risk in an exposed population (absolute risk) and the risk in an unexposed population.

Risk: The probability of harm being caused.

Serious Adverse Events (or, Serious Adverse Drug Reaction): A serious adverse event or reaction is any untoward medical occurrence that at any dose: results in death, hospitalization or prolongation of hospitalization, persistent or significant disability or incapacity, life threatening, a congenital anomaly or birth defect. [The two terminologies serious and severe often cause confusion and are not synonymous. They cannot be used interchangeably. Severe describes the intensity (severity) of an event and the event may be minor medical significance (severe headache). On the other hand, seriousness (not severity) refers the outcome of the event on the patient].

Side Effect: Any unintended effect of a medicine occurring at doses normally used in human which is related to pharmacological properties of the medicine. But it could be beneficial too.

Signal: Reported information on a possible causal relationship between an adverse event and a drug, the relationship being unknown or incompletely documented previously. Usually more than a single report is necessary to generate a signal, depending on the seriousness of the event and the quality of information.

Spontaneous Report: Unsolicited communication by healthcare professionals or consumers that describes one or more ADRs in a patient who was given one or more medicinal products and that does not derive from a study or any organized data collection scheme.

VigiAccess: Open access to WHO database of suspected adverse drug reactions.

VigiBase: WHO database of individual case safety report.

VigiFlow: Spontaneous reporting data entry and analytical tool for WHO database.

VigiLyze: Powerful search and analysis tool that provide access to WHO database and instantly provides data in graph and table format.

VigiMed: Forum that provides access to safety concern in other countries [WHO Programme].

VigiMine: Data Mining tool as a part of VigiSearch.

VigiSearch: Search tool for searching VigiBase database.

Websites of Interest and Some Important References

1. Asian Pharmacoepidemiology Network: http://www.aspennet.asia/
2. Australian Prescriber: http://www.australianprescriber.com/
3. Central Drug Standard Control Organization: http://cdsco.nic.in/pharmacovigilance.htm
4. Council for international Organization of Medical Sciences: http://www.cioms.ch/
5. Current Challenges in Pharmacovigilance: Pragmatic Approaches, Report of CIOMS Working Group V, CIOMS, Geneva, 2001.
6. Guru Prasad Mohanta, Textbook on Clinical Research: A Guide for Aspiring Professionals and Professionals, PharmaMed Press, 2011.
7. International Conference on Harmonization of Technical Requirements for Registration of Pharmaceuticals for Human Use: http://www.ich.org/
8. International Society for Pharmacoepidemiology: https://www.pharmacoepi.org/
9. International Society of Pharmacovigilance: http://www.isoponline.org/
10. Management of Safety Information from Clinical Trials, Report of CIOMS Working Group VI, CIOMS, Geneva, 2005.
11. National Pharmacopoeia Commission: http://ipc.nic.in/index1.asp?EncHid=&lang=1&linkid=60&lid=176
12. Patrick Waller, An Introduction to Pharmacovigilance, Wiley – Blackwell, UK, 2010.
13. Pharmacovigilance Toolkit: http://pvtoolkit.org/

14. Raman Sehgal, Rajat Sethi and Shobha Rani Hiremath, Elements of Pharmacovigilance, Kongposh Publication, New Delhi, 2010.
15. Ronald D. Mann and Elizabeth Andrews (Ed), Pharmacovigilance, Second Edition, John Wiley & Sons Limited, England, 2007.
16. S. K. Gupta (Ed), Textbook of Pharmacovigilance, Jaypee Brothers Medical Publishers (P) Ltd., New Delhi, 2011.
17. Safety of Medicines, World Health Organization, Geneva, 2002.
18. Society of Pharmacovigilance, India: https://www.facebook.com/SOPI.India/
19. The Importance of Pharmacovigilance, World Health Organization, 2002.
20. The Uppsala Monitoring Centre: http://www.who-umc.org/
21. Uppsala Reports: http://www.who-umc.org/DynPage.aspx?id=105825&mn1=7347&mn2=7259&mn3=7297&mn4=7494
22. View Point – Part 1, the Uppsala Monitoring Centre, 2002.
23. View Point – Part 2, the Uppsala Monitoring Centre, 2005.
24. WHO Collaborating Centre for Advocacy and Training in Pharmacovigilance: http://www.who-pvafrica.org/index.php/pharmacovigilance
25. WHO Pharmaceuticals Newsletter: http://www.who.int/medicines/publications/newsletter/en/
26. WHO Policy Perspectives on Medicines – Pharmacovigilance: ensuring the safe use of medicines, WHO, October 2004.
27. World Health Organization: http://www.who.int/medicines/areas/quality_safety/safety_efficacy/pharmvigi/en/index.html

Index

9 789352 301034

Printed at Repro India Ltd.